# Trends in Andrology and Sexual Medicine

**Series Editors**

Emmanuele A. Jannini
Chair of Endocrinology & Medical Sexology (ENDOSEX),
Department of Systems Medicine
University of Rome Tor Vergata
Rome, Italy

Carlo Foresta
Chair of Endocrinology, Department of Medicine, Unit of Andrology
and Reproductive Medicine
University of Padua
Padova, Italy

Andrea Lenzi
Chair of Endocrinology, Department of Experimental Medicine,
Section of Medical Pathophysiology, Food Science and Endocrinology
Sapienza University of Rome
Rome, Rome, Italy

Mario Maggi
Chair of Endocrinology, Department of Experimental, Clinical
and Biomedical Sciences, Andrology and Sexual Medicine Unit
University of Florence
Florence, Italy

This series will serve as a comprehensive and authoritative resource that presents state of the art knowledge and practice within the fields of Andrology and Sexual Medicine, covering basic science and clinical and psychological aspects. Each volume will focus on a specific topic relating to reproductive or sexual health, such as male and female sexual disorders (from erectile dysfunction to vaginismus, and from hypoactive desire to ejaculatory disturbances), diagnostic issues in infertility and sexual dysfunction, and current and emerging therapies (from assisted reproduction techniques to testosterone supplementation, and from PDE5i to SSRIs for premature ejaculation). In addition, selected new topics not previously covered in a single monograph will be addressed, examples including male osteoporosis and the approach of traditional Chinese medicine to sexual medicine. Against the background of rapid progress in Andrology and Sexual Medicine, the series will meet the need of readers for detailed updates on new discoveries in physiology and pathophysiology and in the therapy of human sexual and reproductive disorders.

More information about this series at http://www.springer.com/series/13846

Donatella Paoli • Francesco Lombardo
Andrea Lenzi

# Atlas of Human Semen Examination

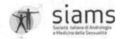

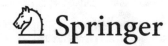

Donatella Paoli
Department of Experimental Medicine
Sapienza University of Rome
Rome
Italy

Francesco Lombardo
Department of Experimental Medicine
Sapienza University of Rome
Rome
Italy

Andrea Lenzi
Department of Experimental Medicine
Sapienza University of Rome
Rome
Italy

ISSN 2367-0088             ISSN 2367-0096   (electronic)
Trends in Andrology and Sexual Medicine
ISBN 978-3-030-40000-2      ISBN 978-3-030-39998-6   (eBook)
https://doi.org/10.1007/978-3-030-39998-6

This Springer imprint is published by the registered company Springer Nature Switzerland AG
The registered company address is: Gewerbestrasse 11, 6330 Cham, Switzerland

# Preface

This new editorial venture by Springer is, necessarily, dedicated in its entirety to Loredana Gandini. Everything in this volume speaks of her: her initial idea, her hard work under the microscope taking the photos, the long hours she spent choosing the best images, the graphic design of the cover... Loredana did all this with the skill, scientific expertise, dedication and joy that characterized her entire scientific life.

We will never forget how her face lit up when the first edition of the *Atlante di Seminologia* was published in 1999, nor her immense satisfaction at its success—which prompted the publication of a second edition in 2010, for which the title was changed to *Diagnostica per immagini dello spermatozoo umano* ["Diagnostic imaging of human spermatozoa"]. This very success was the fruit of her tenacity in tracking down the clearest and most educational images for the readers. We will always remember the many hours we spent discussing the best shots and the right magnification for her beloved *goni*, *citi*, *tidi* and *zoi*, as she called them.

Sadly, Loredana's life was cut cruelly short before she could see the English edition of her labour of love, but we are still gratified by the great interest that this volume continues to arouse; this gives us the motivation and enthusiasm to continue building upon her remarkable achievement.

Rome, Italy

Donatella Paoli
Andrea Lenzi
Francesco Lombardo

# Contents

# Introduction

This volume is divided into two main parts. The first consists of a large collection of images of the main abnormal sperm forms and non-sperm cellular elements found in semen, including a short section dedicated to the basic concepts of spermatogenesis and structure of the male gamete: a reference to be kept by the microscope at all times. Seminal fluid examinations are all too often performed after only the most basic of training, as if they were a non-specialist analysis. There is a clear need to combine an objective cytomorphological evaluation with a functional interpretation, in order to assess the semen's fertilizing potential.

The interpretation above all of sperm morphology has varied so much over time that it is almost impossible to compare results from different retrospective studies and laboratories. This poor comparability also makes it difficult to properly diagnose and treat infertile patients. However, an adequate morphological evaluation, even under an optical microscope, can enable the identification of pathological monomorphisms that lead to congenital forms (e.g. Globozoospermia); these can then be subsequently confirmed using electron microscopy. No less important from both a diagnostic and speculative perspective is the identification of "round cells"—i.e. all cells present in the semen that are not mature gametes.

In relation to immature germ cells, our group has produced a number of articles (Gandini et al., Hum. Reprod., 14: 1022, 1999; Salanova M. et al., Lab. Invest. 79: 1127, 1999) for which the correct identification and selection of the germ cells present in the semen were essential. The identification of germ cells is particularly important in cases of azoospermia (subsequently confirmed with seminal biochemistry data), as a marker of the patency of the seminal tract, or as a response to gonadotropin therapy in patients with hypogonadotropic hypogonadism. The selection of germ cells is also a fundamental step for the most advanced genetic and molecular studies aiming to shed light on the still unsolved problems of human spermatogenesis.

The second part of this new volume concerns the evaluation of sperm chromatin integrity with TUNEL, one of the most commonly used methods in andrological research. It includes a description of the chromatin molecular structure and possible causes of nuclear fragmentation, as well as numerous images to aid the understanding and interpretation of the cellular signs induced by chromatin fragmentation. The study of sperm DNA damage is particularly relevant in an era when assisted reproductive techniques are widely used, leading to a need for a predictive test of success in terms of fertilization, embryo quality and implantation. Several studies in the literature have demonstrated high levels of sperm DNA damage in men with severe spermatogenetic disorders, while others have found that

© Springer Nature Switzerland AG 2020
D. Paoli et al., *Atlas of Human Semen Examination*, Trends in Andrology and Sexual Medicine,
https://doi.org/10.1007/978-3-030-39998-6_1

DNA fragmentation has a negative impact on the outcome of both natural and assisted fertilization. Numerous efforts have been made in recent years to identify a suitable test that evaluates sperm DNA integrity, although the clinical significance of such a test has not yet been established.

## 1 Notes on Human Spermatogenesis

Spermatogenesis is a process involving the proliferation and differentiation of undifferentiated stem cells into spermatozoa. It takes place in the seminiferous tubules of the testis and is divided into three sequential phases: proliferation of spermatogonia, meiosis and spermiogenesis.

The proliferative phase takes place in the basal lamina of the seminiferous tubules. The clonal expansion of the spermatogonia in this phase allows both the production of germ cells destined to become primary spermatocytes (the first step of the spermatogenetic process) and the maintenance of a pool of stem cells. Spermatogonia are classified as type A, which may be dark (Ad, with dispersed, intensely coloured chromatin) or pale (Ap, with finely dispersed, weakly coloured chromatin), and type B. Following mitotic division, during differentiation type Ad spermatogonia produce both type Ap and further undifferentiated type Ad spermatogonia; the latter constitute the reserve of stem cells necessary for subsequent multiplication and differentiation cycles. Mitotic division of type Ap gives rise to type B spermatogonia; further mitosis produces primary spermatocytes (preleptotene) which, after duplicating their DNA, undergo the first meiotic division. There is no further development of germ cells until the beginning of puberty, when serum levels of gonadotropins and androgens rise and spermatogenetic activity resumes.

The prophase of the first meiotic division is rather long. It is characterized by a progressive increase in the size of the nuclei of the primary tetraploid spermatocytes and by the genetic recombination of the homologous chromosomes. It can be divided into five stages: leptotene, zygotene, pachytene, diplotene and diakinesis. In the leptotene stage, the chromosomes, consisting of two sister chromatids, appear as thin tangled filaments. During the zygotene stage, the homologous chromosomes appear to form the synaptonemal complex. In the pachytene stage the chromosomes shorten and thicken and DNA is exchanged between homologous chromosomes, the so-called crossing over; in this phase the cell size increases, and the pachytene spermatocyte is therefore the largest cell of the germ line. During the diplotene stage, the synaptonemal complex disappears and the chromosomes separate—except in the chiasm region, the area where the exchange of genetic material took place. In the final phase, diakinesis, the chromosomes condense.

The cells then proceed through the metaphase, in which the two centromeres of each bivalent align on the equatorial plate, and the anaphase, in which they separate and migrate to the opposite poles of the cell. In the telophase, the final stage of the first meiotic division, cytodieresis, takes place, leading to the formation of two daughter

© Springer Nature Switzerland AG 2020
D. Paoli et al., *Atlas of Human Semen Examination*, Trends in Andrology and Sexual Medicine,
https://doi.org/10.1007/978-3-030-39998-6_2

cells. It is interesting to note that cytodieresis of the germ cells, i.e. the separation of the cytoplasm at the end of cell division, is incomplete; the germ cells derived from a common spermatogonium thus remain in a syncytium (connected by cytoplasmic bridges) until the mature germ cells are released for spermiation. This syncytial structure allows the germ cells to "communicate" and coordinate their development synchronously. The two haploid daughter cells derived from the first meiotic division are called secondary spermatocytes.

Between the first and the second meiotic divisions there is a very short interphase in which no DNA is synthesized. The second meiotic division process begins almost immediately thereafter, and secondary spermatocytes progress from the prophase to telophase. The second meiotic division involves the separation of the sister chromatids along the centromere; at the end of this process, each secondary spermatocyte is divided and the daughter cells, called spermatids, contain a haploid genome. By the end of meiosis, each primary spermatocyte has thus split twice, giving rise to four spermatids.

Spermatids are initially round cells that are completely different from mature spermatozoa. They undergo a series of gradual modifications known as spermiogenesis, which transforms them into flagellated elongated cells with independent movement—spermatozoa. This transformation occurs through four successive phases, known as the Golgi, cap, acrosome and maturation phases.

In the Golgi phase, proacrosomal granules rich in carbohydrates (detectable by the periodic Schiff acid reaction, specific for polysaccharides) appear in the Golgi body and fuse into a single acrosomal granule. The cap phase involves the expansion of the membrane limiting the acrosomal vesicle, which reaches around the front two-thirds of the nucleus to form the so-called acrosome cap. At the same time, the centrioles migrate to the pole opposite the acrosome formation, where the distal centriole gives rise to the flagellum.

In the acrosome phase, considerable variations take place in the structures of the acrosome, nucleus and flagellum. The acrosomal granule widens until it fills the entire cap, the nucleus lengthens and migrates to the cell periphery, and the nuclear chromatin condenses into coarse grains. The cytoplasm moves towards the caudal pole of the nucleus and wraps around the proximal part of the flagellum, where the mitochondria are arranged like a sleeve.

Finally, in the maturation phase the spermatozoon assumes its final form. The nucleus becomes a compact, homogeneous structure, the tail undergoes its final differentiations and the excess cytoplasm is eliminated, and will subsequently constitute the so-called residual bodies that will be engulfed by the Sertoli cells.

As the cells progress through the spermiogenetic process, they are pushed by the tubular fluid towards the lumen of the seminiferous tubules, culminating in the release of mature spermatozoa into the lumen (spermiation). In humans, the entire process, from spermatogonium to mature sperm, takes about 72 days.

This process requires complex interactions between germ cells and the somatic cells in the seminiferous tubules, called Sertoli cells. These are large, coarsely cylindrical cells that do not divide; they go from the basal lamina to the lumen of the seminiferous tubule and wrap the cells of the spermatogenetic process (with the exception of spermatogonia, which rest directly on the basement membrane) through a complicated intertwining of cytoplasmic extensions. The cytoplasmic prolongations of the various Sertoli cells are interconnected by narrow junctions and constitute the so-called blood-testicular barrier, ensuring the specific microenvironment required for the correct development of germ cells inside the seminiferous tubules. The Sertoli cells offer a decisive contribution to this microenvironment by producing proteins and hormones and secreting paracrine factors that enable the exchange of information between germ and support cells and between peritubular and interstitial cells.

# 2 Morphological Structure of the Spermatozoon

Under an optical microscope the mature human spermatozoon appears to consist of a flattened oval apical portion, called the "head", a short neck and a long, thin flagellum, called the "tail". The head is formed by two domains, the nucleus and the acrosome. The compact nucleus contains condensed DNA with a haploid chromosomal structure and is two-third covered by the acrosomal complex. This cap-shaped structure consists of an internal acrosomal membrane in contact with the nuclear membrane and an external acrosome membrane positioned below the plasma membrane.

The acrosome, which derives from the spermatid's Golgi body, contains lytic enzymes—essential for oocyte penetration. The plasma membrane surrounding the acrosome and nucleus typically has a trilaminar appearance under the electron microscope, with a thick glycoprotein coating (sperm coating substances) on the external surface.

The short (just 1 micron) neck extends from the posterior part of the nuclear membrane to the point where the intermediate segment of the tail joins the head. The tail consists of the axial or axonemal filamentous complex, composed of a pair of microtubules located centrally and nine pairs arranged at the periphery (9 + 2 organization). This complex of filaments runs along the entire length of the tail, which is divided into an "intermediate segment" 5–6 μ long, a "main segment" about 45 μ long and a "final segment" about 5 μ long. In the intermediate segment the complex is surrounded by nine dense external fibres, which are thin where they are in contact with the microtubules and become thicker as they approach the external surface. These in turn are surrounded (in the intermediate segment only) by the mitochondrial sheath, essential for sperm respiration and for the production of energy. The intermediate segment is separated from the main segment by a structure called the annulus, a ring of dense material that adheres to the flagellum membrane.

In the main segment, the axoneme and external fibres are surrounded by a fibrous sheath composed of two columns of dense fibres. This fibrous sheath terminates abruptly at the junction between the main and terminal segments; the terminal segment itself is constituted by the axoneme covered by the plasma membrane alone.

Sperm morphology is evaluated fresh at 400× and on stained smears at 1000×. Numerous morphological classifications have been proposed. The WHO's current classification is as follows (2010):

**Oval head: normal**

**Head defects**
- large (macrocephalia)
- small (microcephalia)
- amorphous
- tapered
- pyriform
- round (no acrosome; small)
- vacuolated
- double head
- pinhead
- small or large acrosomal areas

**Neck and midpiece defects**
- bent neck
- asymmetrical insertion of the midpiece into the head
- thick insertion
- thin

**Tail defects**
- short
- looped
- coiled
- bent
- double, multiple
- broken

**Excess residual cytoplasm**

# 3 Non-sperm Cellular Components of the Seminal Fluid

Examination of fresh or stained seminal fluid also reveals any non-sperm cellular components. These may include the following:

- Elements of the spermatogenesis process: any cellular elements produced prior to the spermatozoa may be present:
  - spermatogonia
  - primary spermatocytes
  - secondary spermatocytes
  - spermatids;
- Leukocytes: predominantly:
  - polymorphonuclear leukocytes
  - lymphocytes
  - macrophages;
- Red blood cells;
- Epithelial cells sloughed off from the accessory glands or the urogenital ducts.

## 3.1 Elements from the Spermatogenesis Process

Spermatogonia have little cytoplasm and a round nucleus, with intensely (dark, type Ad) or weakly (pale, type Ap) coloured chromatin and 1 or 2 nucleoli. They are the least common cells in the seminal fluid as they are in direct contact with the basement membrane and are therefore more distant from the lumen of the seminiferous tubule.

Primary spermatocytes are large cells with a large central nucleus in which, rarely, a nucleolus may be seen. The appearance of chromatin depends on its stage of meiotic division; it may be thickened in clods or show a characteristic filament appearance reminiscent of cerebral convolutions.

Binuclear elements deriving from incomplete separation of the cytoplasm are a common finding. The division of spermatogonia and spermatocytes differs from that of somatic cells, due to incomplete cytodieresis. The daughter cells remain connected by intracytoplasmic bridges, which are transient structures in the somatic cells but remain in the seminiferous epithelium until the final phase of spermatid differentiation into spermatozoa.

Secondary spermatocytes are small round cells with a central thickened core. They derive from the first meiotic division and remain in the interphase for a very short period, and so are rarely found in seminal fluid.

The morphology of spermatids depends on their stage of maturation. Types a and b are small, round cells with a central thickened nucleus characterized by a granular chromatin and with a cytoplasm rich in proacrosomal granules deriving from the Golgi body. Types c and d are elongated cells characterized by an eccentric nucleus with a more condensed chromatin.

As the maturation progresses the proacrosomal granules merge into a single granule to form the acrosome, the chromatin is further compacted and the cytoplasm is reduced to take on a wake-like appearance. At this point the spermatid has assumed the morphological characteristics of the spermatozoon. Spermatids and primary spermatocytes are the elements from the spermatogenesis process most commonly found in semen.

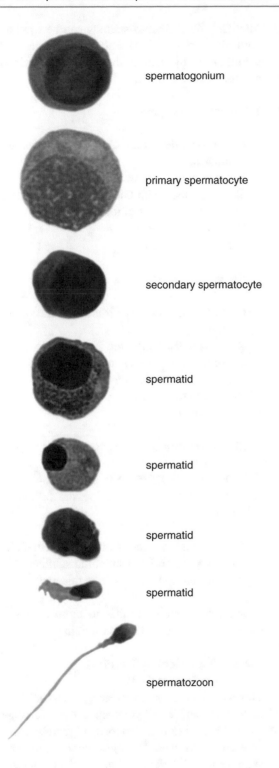

spermatogonium

primary spermatocyte

secondary spermatocyte

spermatid

spermatid

spermatid

spermatid

spermatozoon

# 4    Morphological Study of the Seminal Fluid

Sperm morphology is first performed on fresh semen at 400× during the evaluation of the other semen parameters. A number of slides are then prepared as appropriate for each sample and examined under a 1000× optical microscope. Cytology specimens must be prepared using degreased slides so that the smear is distributed evenly over the entire surface. If the smear tends to retract, the slides should be pre-treated by immersing them in absolute or 95% ethanol to enable more complete adhesion of the sample.

For the morphological evaluation of spermatozoa separated by swim up or of washed spermatozoa, it should be remembered that samples prepared in this way will not produce a perfect smear because they do not contain proteins. In this case, it is advisable to use polylysine-coated slides or to add 1% albumin to the cell suspension.

## 4.1    Preparation of Semen Smears

- Use slides with a frosted edge bearing the patient's name.
- Place a 10 µL drop on the slide at the end of the frosted edge.
- Immerse one end of the coverslip (24 × 32 or 24 × 50 mm) in the drop and let the seminal fluid spread.
- Streak very gently, in order to minimize sperm damage, over the entire length of the slide.
- Allow to air dry.
- Fix the slides in absolute or 95% ethanol or in methanol for 15 minutes.
- Allow to air dry, then stain.

## 4.2    Staining Techniques

### 4.2.1    May-Grünwald-Giemsa Staining
This method uses two dye solutions: Giemsa (blue II-eosin) and May-Grünwald (methylene-eosin blue), both readily available on the market.

May-Grünwald-Giemsa staining can be used on both air-dried and fixed smears; it enables cell identification by staining the nucleus blue-violet and the cytoplasm pink.

1. Procedure for sperm

- Cover the slide in May-Grünwald solution for 4 minutes.
- Rinse with distilled water.
- Cover the slide with Giemsa solution (diluted 1:10 in distilled water) for 15 minutes.
- Rinse with distilled water.
- Air dry, then mount.

2. Procedure for germ cells

- Cover the slide in May-Grünwald solution for 4 minutes.
- Rinse with distilled water.
- Cover the slide with Giemsa solution (diluted 1:20 in distilled water) for 15 minutes.
- Rinse with distilled water.
- Air dry, then mount.

### 4.2.2    Diff Quik Staining for Sperm Cells
Diff Quik (Dade Behring) is a ready-to-use kit that allows rapid staining using the following solutions:

- fixative solution (triarylmethane in methanol);
- staining solution 1 (eosinophilic xanthene);
- staining solution 2 (basophilic thiazine).

It produces stains similar to those achieved using May-Grünwald-Giemsa staining.

### 4.2.3    Papanicolau Staining for Sperm Cells
This technique uses a nuclear dye (Harris' haematoxylin) and two cytoplasmic dyes [Orange G6 and EA-50 (eosin-alcohol)], all readily available on the market. The dyes work together to stain the nuclei dark grey-blue and the cytoplasm pink or orange.

# 5 Chromatin Aspect

## 5.1 Chromatin Organization in Human Sperm

Male infertility is diagnosed on the basis of light microscope assessment of various sperm parameters such as concentration, motility and morphology, which are important markers of semen quality. However, quantitative and qualitative sperm analysis is only part of the story: sperm chromatin and DNA integrity are also essential for the fertilization and normal development of the embryo. During spermiogenesis—the last stage of spermatogenesis, in which the round spermatid transforms into the mature spermatozoon—there are major reorganizations of the genome, in addition to these morphological changes. Protamines, which are arginine-rich species-specific proteins expressed only in males, have a fundamental role in this phase.

The term protamine was originally coined by Friedrich Miescher in 1874, referring to an organic base associated with the "nuclein" of the Rhine salmon sperm nucleus. Protamines are the most abundant proteins in the sperm nucleus and are found nowhere else. Sperm DNA is strongly bound to protamines, taking on a highly compact toroidal structure. DNA–protamine interaction takes place between the arginine domains in the protamines and the phosphodiester DNA skeleton. Packaging of the sperm nucleus involves the progressive substitution of somatic and testicular histones with protamines, although about 15% of human sperm DNA remains bound to the histone fraction. Recent studies have demonstrated that the histones bound to DNA in the sperm cells are associated with gene families with an important role in embryonic differentiation and development. It is thought that the histone fraction may be involved in the reprogramming of the male genome during sperm nuclear decondensation, as well as acting in the paternal imprinting mechanism after fertilization.

The histone/protamine transition mechanism is highly complex and finely regulated. In this phase, arginine- and lysine-rich proteins called transition proteins (TNPs) bind the DNA, thus maintaining an intermediate structure in the protamine deposition sites and facilitating histone elimination. At the end of the spermatogenic process the TNPs are removed and progressively substituted with protamines, whose high cysteine content determines chromatin compaction through the formation of inter- and intramolecular disulphide bridges.

One of the causes of male infertility is changes in the sperm nucleus linked to sperm chromatin abnormalities and protamination defects. Physiological and environmental stress factors, genetic mutations and chromosome abnormalities can modify the complex biochemical processes taking place during spermatogenesis, with negative effects on the chromatin structure and fertility. For example, oxidative stress can induce sperm chromatin fragmentation. Abnormalities like these can also arise during spermiogenesis, following topoisomerase II repair errors. High topoisomerase II levels and DNA strand breaks may be normal in elongated spermatids, possibly as a result of the need to relax the tension caused by the intense torsional movements that the DNA undergoes during nuclear condensation. In this case, the strand breaks are due to a physiological need and do not have any negative consequences if they are then repaired by topoisomerase II before the completion of spermiogenesis. However, if the repair capacity of topoisomerase II is affected or blocked by exposure to inhibitors, the strand breaks might not be repaired perfectly.

Sperm DNA damage has a multifactorial aetiology and can be traced to both endogenous and environmental testicular and post-testicular factors. The latest theory is that sperm DNA damage is caused by altered protamine expression, the excessive production of oxygen free radicals or an apoptotic process. Apoptosis is a form of cell death based on a genetic mechanism that induces a number of cellular, morphological and biochemical changes, resulting in the cell's "suicide". Morphologically, apoptotic cells are characterized by an altered cell skeleton. The chromatin becomes pyknotic and accumulates against the nuclear membrane (chromatin marginalization), giving rise to cellular appearances that have inspired various definitions (half-moon, horseshoe, sickle, etc.) for over a century. Biochemically, one of the most important features of apoptosis is activation of calcium/magnesium-dependent endonucleases. These fragment the cell DNA in a specific manner into nucleosome units of approximately 185 bp. The apoptotic process has also been associated with regulation of the differentiation and maturation processes that lead to the mature sperm. Spermatogonial clonal expansion is in fact decidedly excessive, necessitating a mechanism that can combat this growth in line with the number of Sertoli cells. The inefficiency of human spermatogenesis is well documented: a primary spermatocyte gives rise to just two spermatids, instead of the four that could be theoretically predicted.

Sperm nuclear integrity can be investigated using various methods. The most common is TUNEL, which is based on the use of an enzyme, terminal deoxynucleotide transferase (TdT), which catalyses the polymerization of fluorescein-labelled nucleotides to the 3′-OH terminal end of the fragmented DNA.

The study of sperm DNA damage is particularly important in light of the now widespread use of assisted reproductive technology (ART), and there is an ongoing hunt for a test that can predict success in terms of fertilization, embryo quality and implantation. There have been numerous efforts in recent years to identify a suitable test that evaluates sperm DNA damage. However, the clinical significance of such tests has yet to be established. Numerous studies have used TUNEL to demonstrate nuclear fragmentation in sperm from both infertile patients and patients with andrological and neoplastic diseases (*Gandini et al. Hum. Reprod.,15:830, 2000*). These studies indicate that fragmentation in sperm could be the result of various pathogens or of dysregulation of the spermatogenesis control system. Other studies have correlated sperm fragmentation with reproductive outcome, especially with a reduced pregnancy rate and increased risk of abortion in ART. It should be remembered that the final effect on reproductive success depends not only on the type and magnitude of sperm DNA damage but also on the capacity of the oocyte to repair this damage. The biological effects of an abnormal chromatin structure depend, in fact, on the combination of both the level of sperm chromatin damage and the quality of the oocyte.

## Further Reading

- Danis RB, Samplaski MK (2019) Sperm Morphology: History, Challenges, and Impact on Natural and Assisted Fertility. Curr Urol Rep. 20(8):43
- Gatimel N, Moreau J, Parinaud J, Léandri RD (2017) Sperm morphology: assessment, pathophysiology, clinical relevance, and state of the art in 2017. Andrology. 5(5):845–862
- Neto FT, Bach PV, Najari BB, Li PS, Goldstein M (2016) Spermatogenesis in humans and its affecting factors. Semin Cell Dev Biol. 59:10–26
- Ricci G, Andolfi L, Zabucchi G, Luppi S, Boscolo R, Martinelli M, Zweyer M, Trevisan E (2015) Ultrastructural Morphology of Sperm from Human Globozoospermia. Biomed Res Int. 2015:798754
- Shiraishi K, Matsuyama H (2017) Gonadotropin actions on spermatogenesis and hormonal therapies for spermatogenic disorders. Endocr J. 64(2):123–131
- World Health Organization (2010) WHO laboratory manual for the Examination and processing of human semen, 5th edn. Switzerland, Geneva

# Image Gallery: Sperm Morphology
(Figs. 1–123)

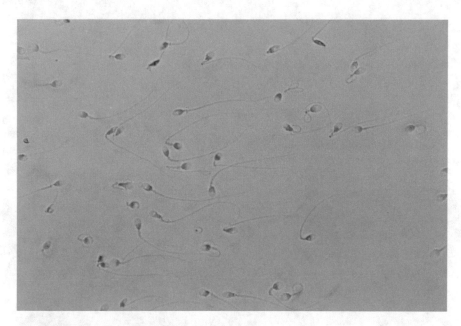

**Fig. 1** Sperm morphological evaluation, unstained
*Unstained 400×*

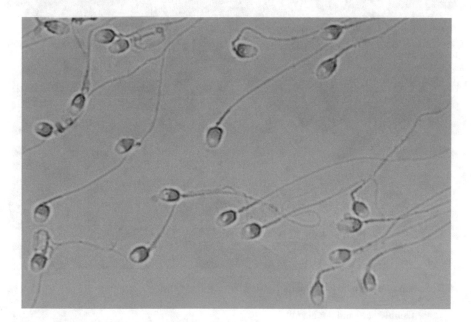

**Fig. 2** Sperm morphological evaluation, unstained
*Unstained 1000×*

© Springer Nature Switzerland AG 2020
D. Paoli et al., *Atlas of Human Semen Examination*, Trends in Andrology and Sexual Medicine,
https://doi.org/10.1007/978-3-030-39998-6_3

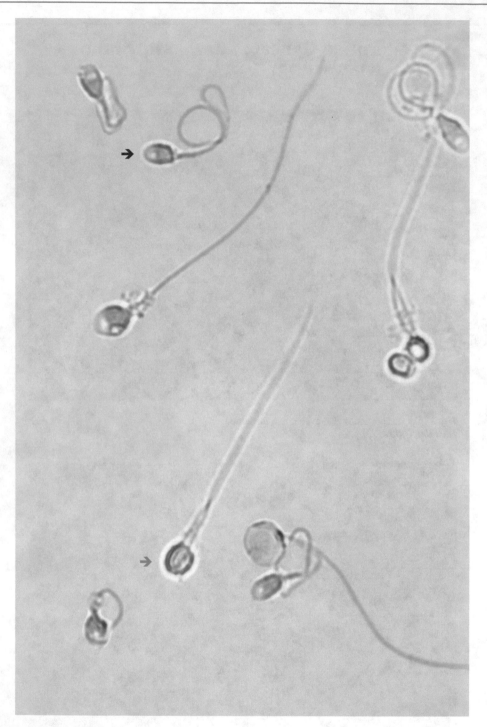

**Fig. 3**  Sperm morphological evaluation, unstained
➜ Small head,
➜ Double head and double tail
*Unstained 1000×*

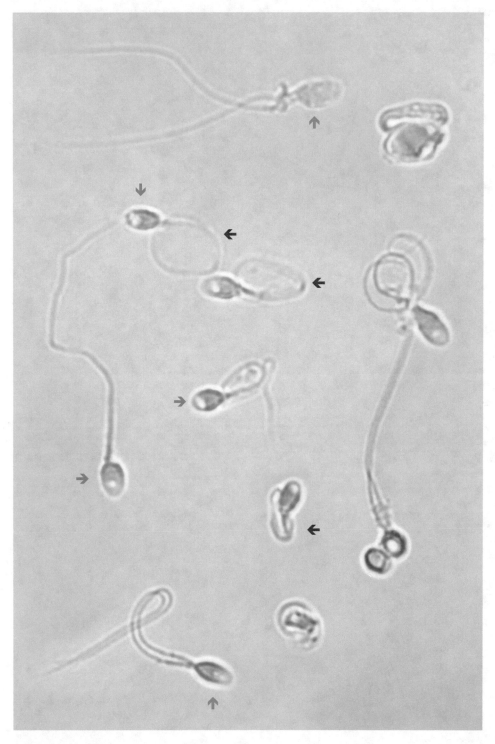

**Fig. 4** Sperm morphological evaluation, unstained
➜ Small head,
➜ Looped tails,
➜ Double tails
*Unstained 1000×*

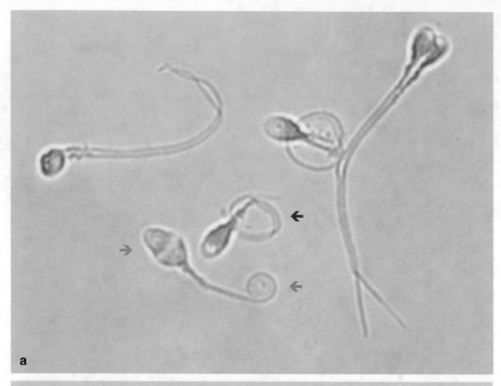

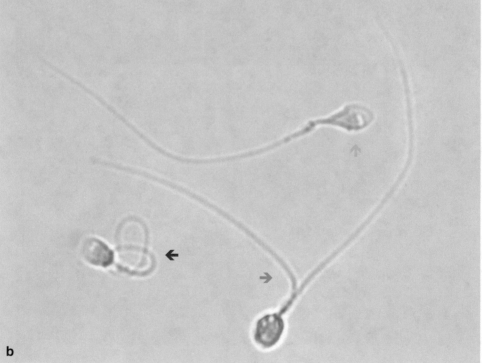

**Fig. 5** Sperm morphological evaluation, unstained
 **a** ➔ Decondensed head, ➔ Looped tail, ➔ Coiled tail
 **b** ➔ Pyriform head, ➔ Double tail, ➔ Coiled tail
*Unstained 1000×*

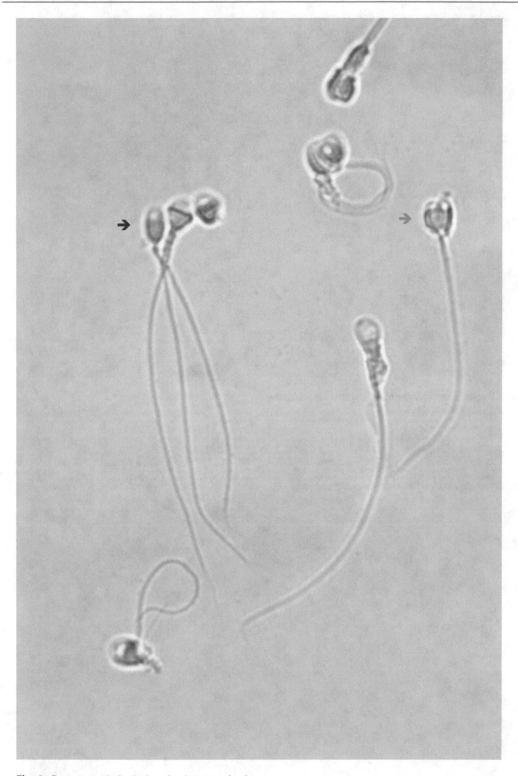

**Fig. 6** Sperm morphological evaluation, unstained
➔ Small head,
➔ Double head
*Unstained 1000×*

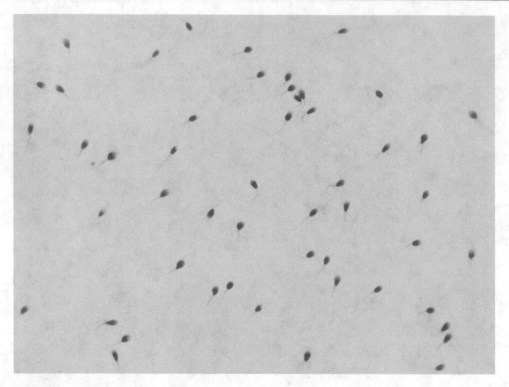

**Fig. 7** Sperm morphological evaluation after staining
*Diff Quik 400×*

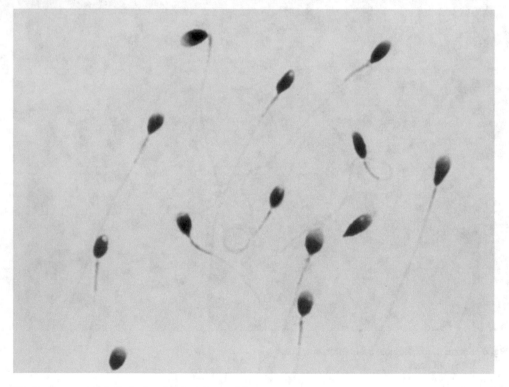

**Fig. 8** Sperm morphological evaluation after staining
*Diff Quik 1000×*

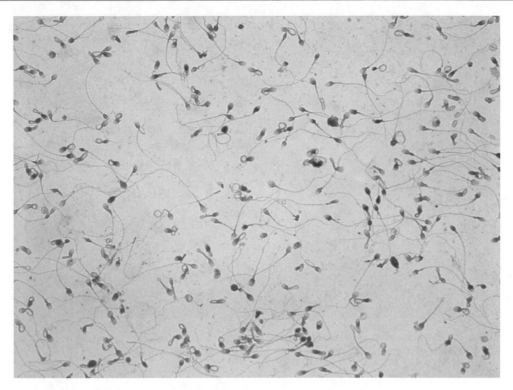

**Fig. 9**  Sperm morphological evaluation after staining
*May-Grünwald-Giemsa 400×*

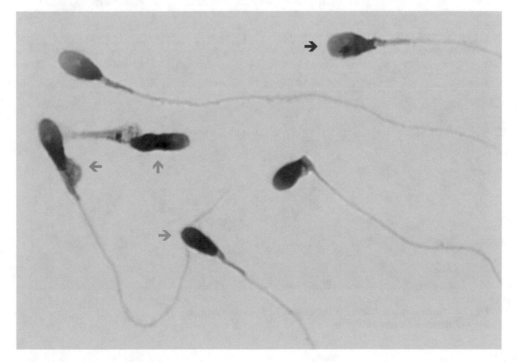

**Fig. 10**  ➔ Amorphous head, ➔ Tapered head, ➔ Excess residual cytoplasm
*May-Grünwald-Giemsa 1000×*

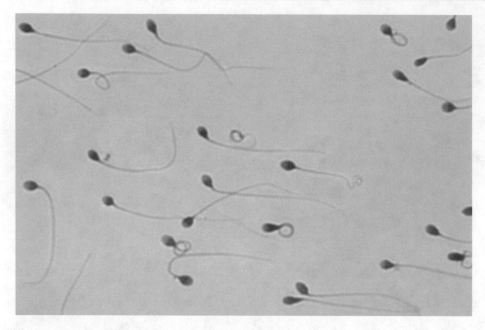

**Fig. 11** Sperm morphological evaluation after staining
*May-Grünwald-Giemsa 500×*

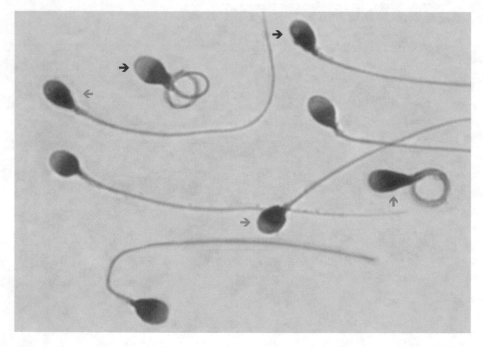

**Fig. 12** ➔ Amorphous heads, ➔ Small heads, ➔ Pyriform head
*May-Grünwald-Giemsa 1000×*

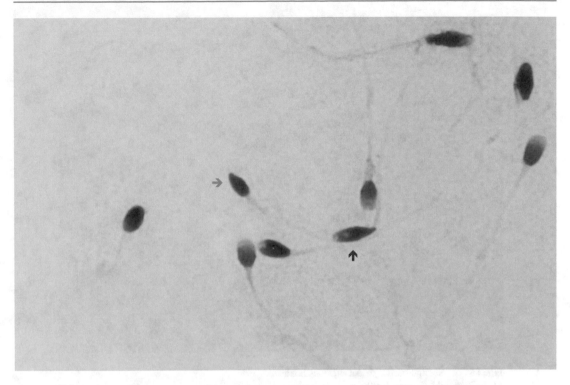

**Fig. 13** ➜ Tapered head and bent neck, ➜ Amorphous head without acrosome
*May-Grünwald-Giemsa 1000×*

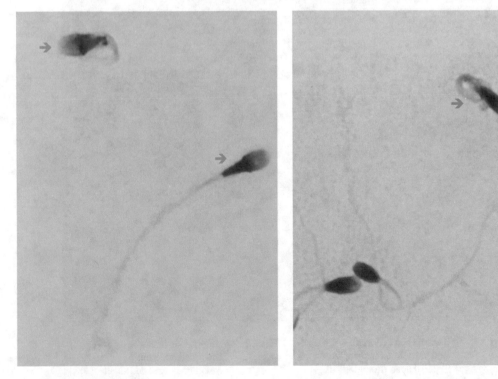

**Fig. 14** ➜ Pyriform heads
*May-Grünwald-Giemsa 1000×*

**Fig. 15** ➜ Tapered head and looped tail
*May-Grünwald-Giemsa 1000×*

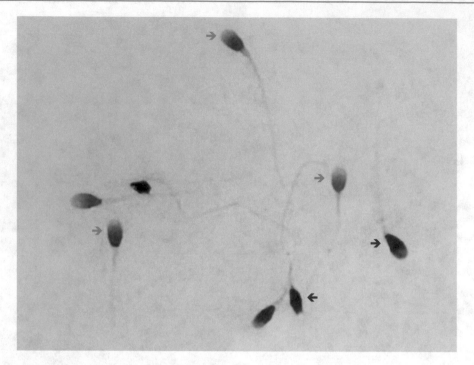

**Fig. 16**  ➔ Normal heads, ➔ Amorphous heads
*May-Grünwald-Giemsa 1000×*

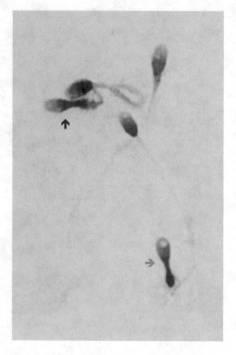

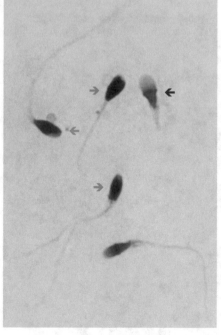

**Fig. 17**  ➔ Tapered head (hourglass-like)
         and vacuolated acrosome,
     ➔ Tapered head (hourglass-like)
*May-Grünwald-Giemsa 1000×*

**Fig. 18**  ➔ Amorphous heads
         and small acrosome
     ➔ Amorphous head and small
         and asymmetrical acrosome,
     ➔ Pyriform head
*May-Grünwald-Giemsa 1000×*

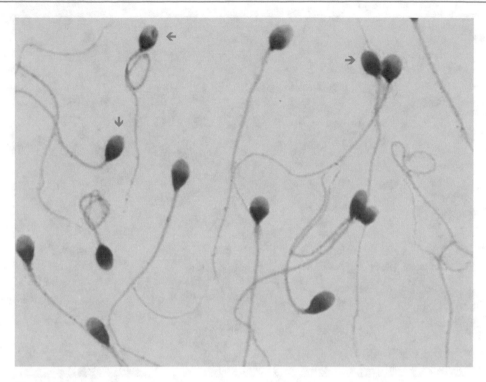

**Fig. 19** ➜ Normal heads
*May-Grünwald-Giemsa 1000×*

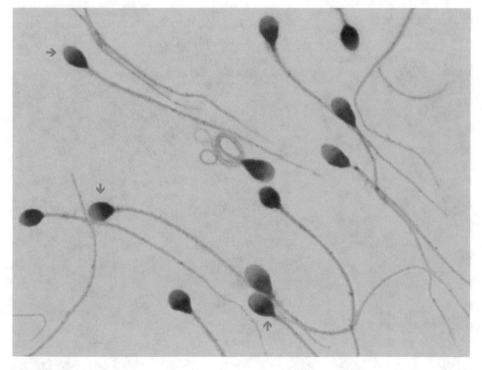

**Fig. 20** ➜ Normal heads
*May-Grünwald-Giemsa 1000×*

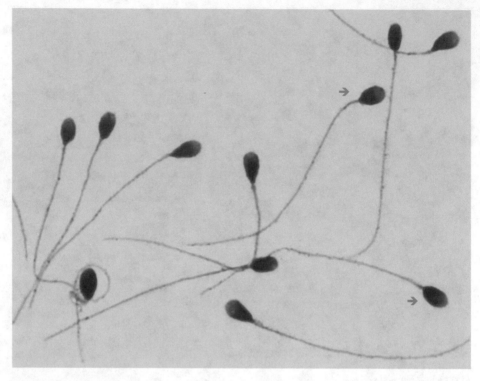

**Fig. 21** ➔ Normal heads
*May-Grünwald-Giemsa 1000×*

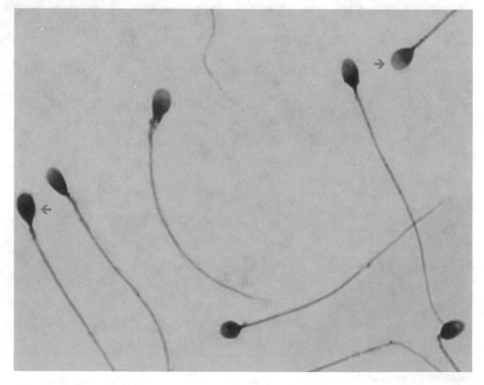

**Fig. 22** ➔ Normal heads
*May-Grünwald-Giemsa 1000×*

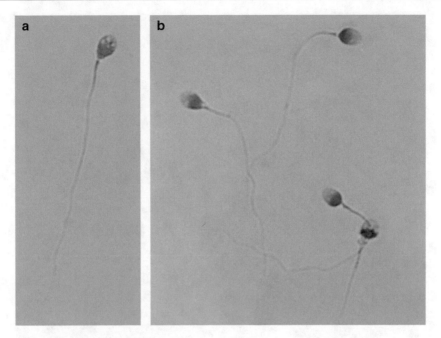

**Fig. 23**  **a**, **b** Vacuoles in acrosomal area
*Papanicolau 1000×*

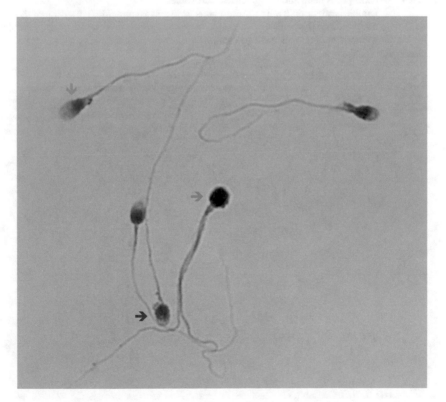

**Fig. 24**  ➔ Round head and double tail, ➔ Amorphous head
➔ Amorphous head and small acrosomal area
*Papanicolau 1000×*

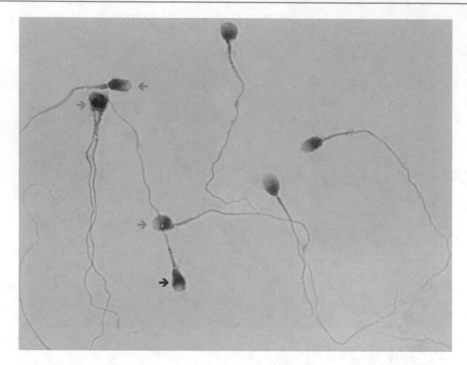

**Fig. 25** ➜ Amorphous head and asymmetrical acrosome,
➜ Double head, double tail ➜ Amorphous head and asymmetrical insertion of the
midpiece into the head
➜ Amorphous head and small acrosome
*Papanicolau 1000×*

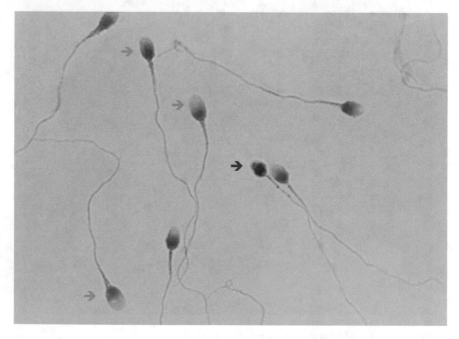

**Fig. 26** ➜ Normal heads, ➜ Small head, ➜ Amorphous head with small acrosome
*Papanicolau 1000×*

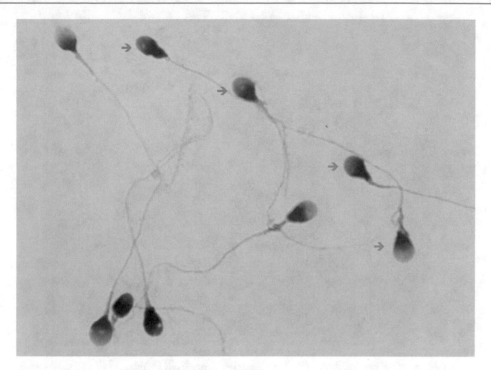

**Fig. 27** ➜ Amorphous heads, ➜ Pyriform heads
*May-Grünwald-Giemsa1000×*

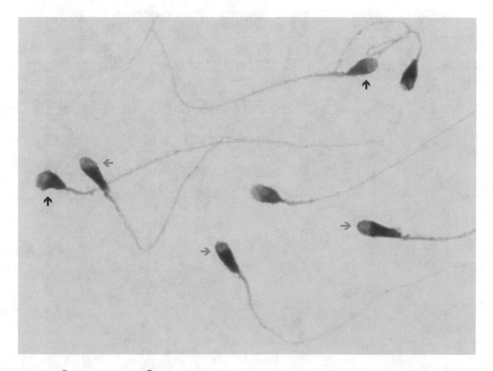

**Fig. 28** ➜ Tapered heads, ➜ Amorphous heads,
*May-Grünwald-Giemsa1000×*

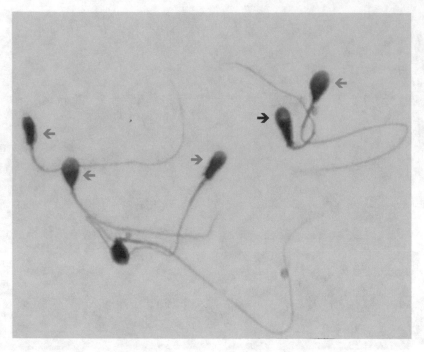

**Fig. 29** ➔ Tapered head, ➔ Pyriform heads, ➔ Amorphous heads
*May-Grünwald-Giemsa 1000×*

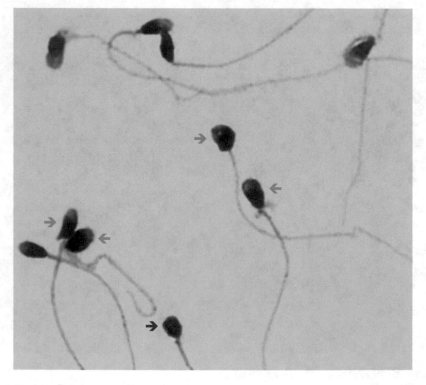

**Fig. 30** ➔ Small head, ➔ Amorphous heads
*May-Grünwald-Giemsa 1000×*

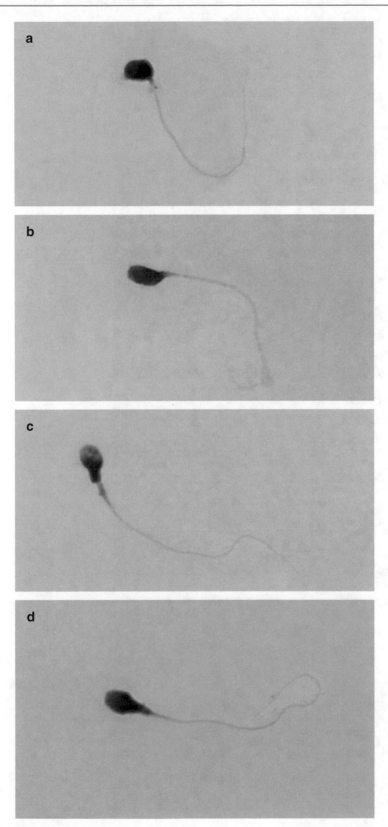

**Fig. 31　a, b, c, d** Amorphous heads
*May-Grünwald-Giemsa1000×*

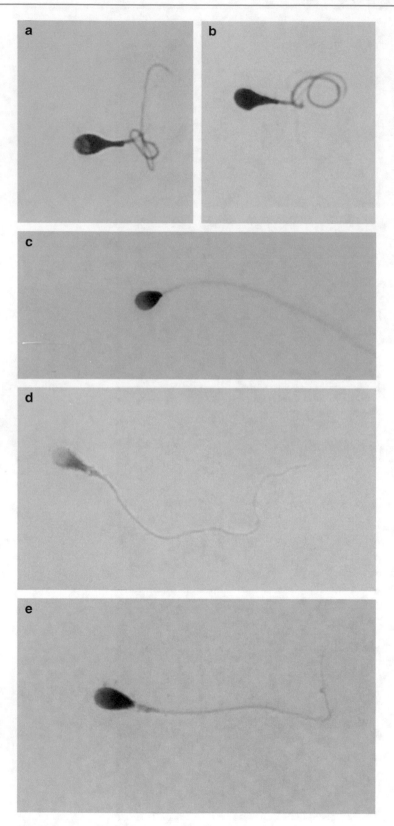

**Fig. 32**  a, b, c, d, e Pyriform heads
*a, b, c, e May-Grünwald-Giemsa1000×, d Papanicolau 1000×*

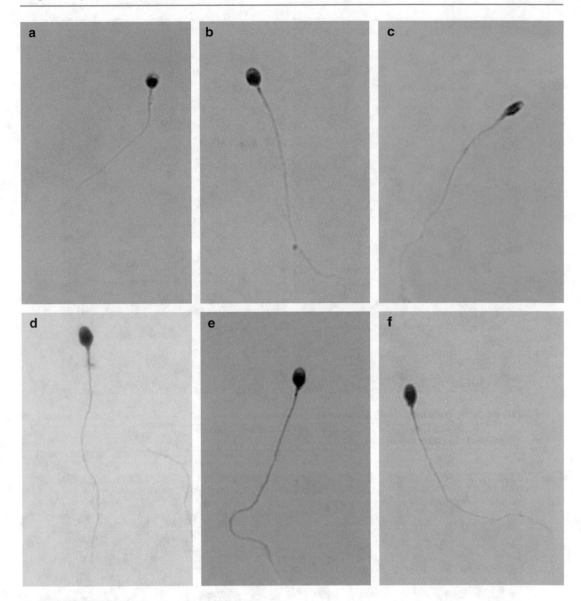

**Fig. 33  a, b, c** Small heads and small acrosome
       **d, e, f** Small heads
*a, b, c Papanicolau 1000×, d, e, f May-Grünwald-Giemsa1000×*

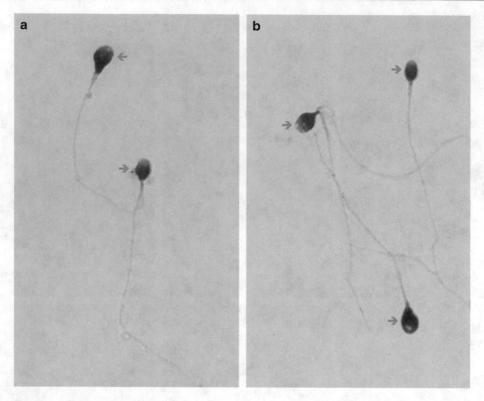

**Fig. 34  a** ➜ Small head, ➜ Pyriform head
      **b** ➜ Small head, ➜ Pyriform heads and vacuolated acrosome
*May-Grünwald-Giemsa1000×*

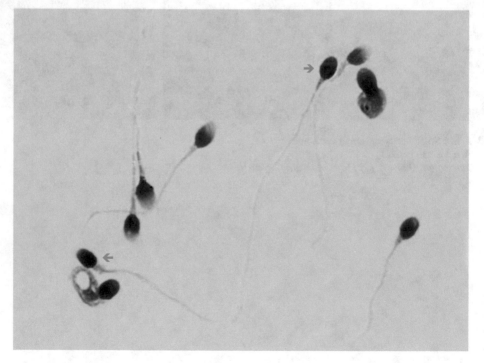

**Fig. 35** ➜ Small heads
*Diff Quik 1000×*

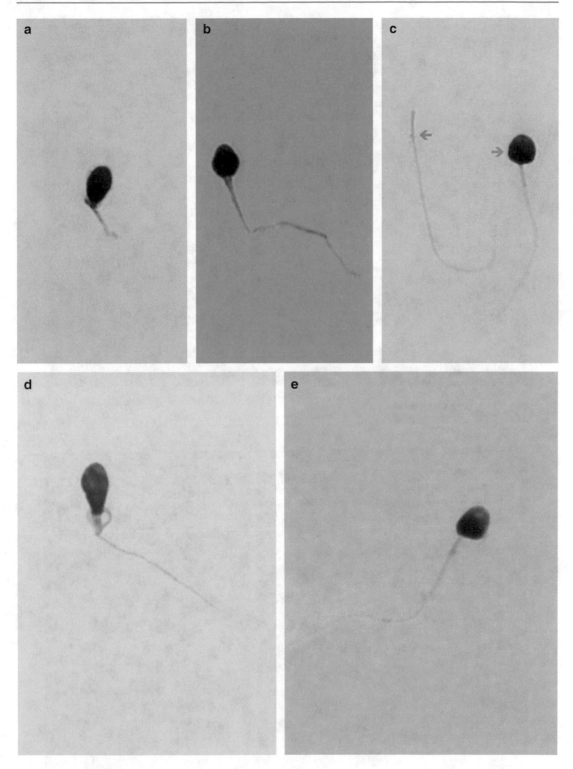

**Fig. 36**  **a** Large head with broken tail
**b** Large head with bent tail
**c** ➔ Pinhead, ➔ Large head
**d, e** Large heads
*May-Grünwald-Giemsa1000×*

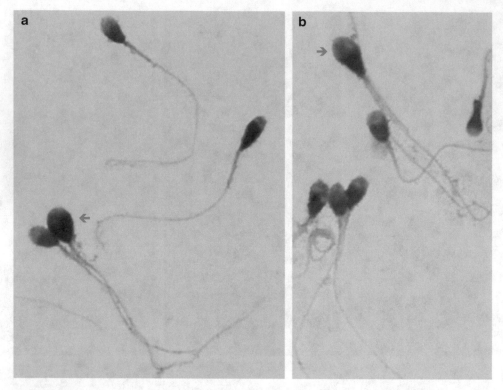

**Fig. 37 a, b →** Large heads
*May-Grünwald-Giemsa1000×*

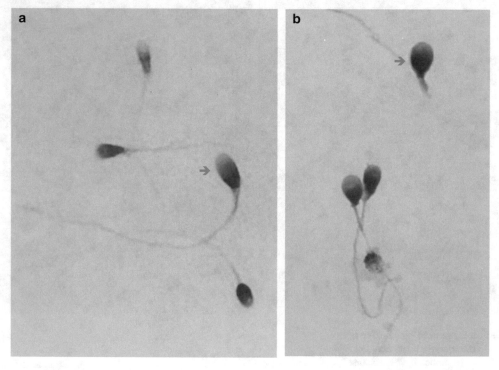

**Fig. 38 a, b →** Large heads
*May-Grünwald-Giemsa1000×*

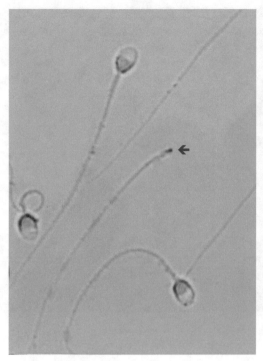

**Fig. 39** ➔ Pinhead
*Unstained 1000×*

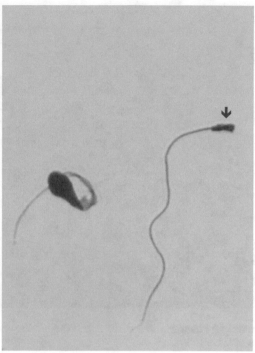

**Fig. 40** ➔ Pinhead
*May-Grünwald-Giemsa1000×*

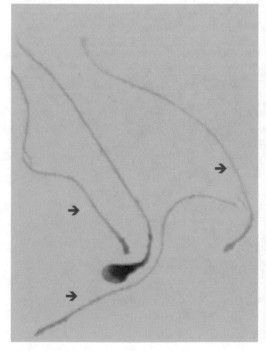

**Fig. 41** ➔ Pinheads
*May-Grünwald-Giemsa1000×*

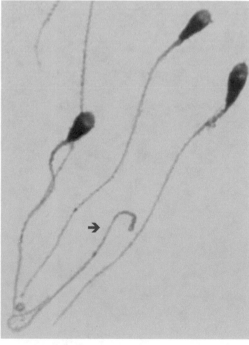

**Fig. 42** ➔ Pinhead
*May-Grünwald-Giemsa1000×*

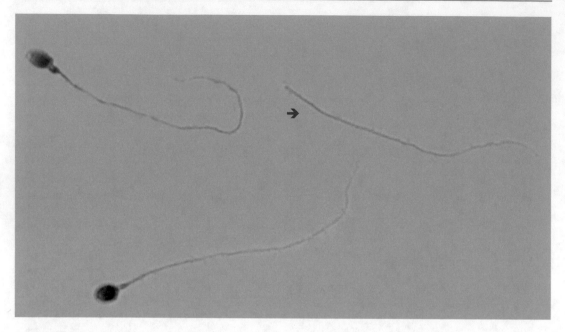

**Fig. 43** ➜ Pinhead
*Papanicolau 1000×*

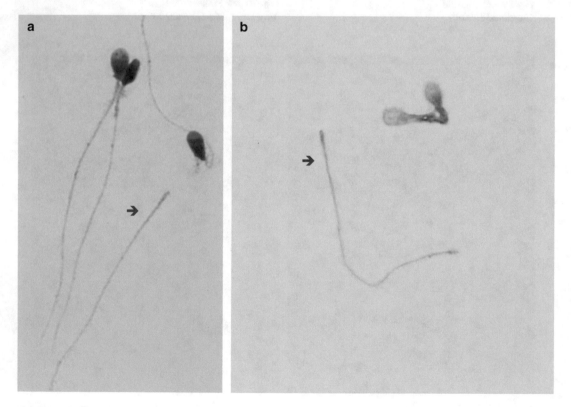

**Fig. 44   a, b** ➜ Pinheads
*a May-Grünwald-Giemsa 1000x, **b** Papanicolau 1000x*

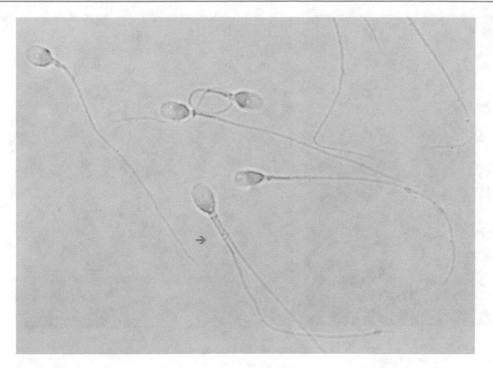

**Fig. 45** ➔ Double tail
*Unstained 1000×*

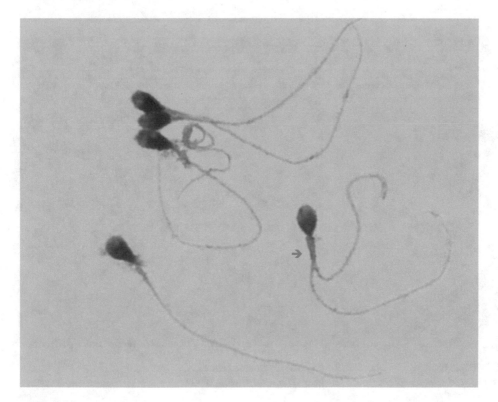

**Fig. 46** ➔ Double tail
*May-Grünwald-Giemsa1000×*

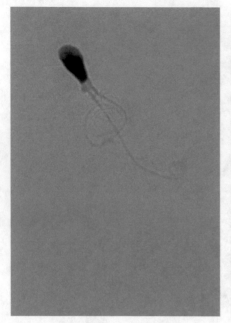

**Fig. 47**  Double tail
*May-Grünwald-Giemsa1000×*

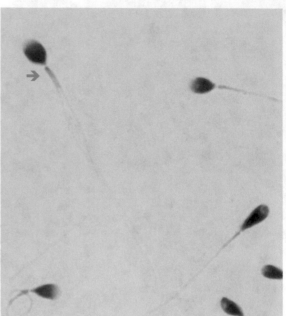

**Fig. 48**  ➔ Double tail
*Diff Quik1000×*

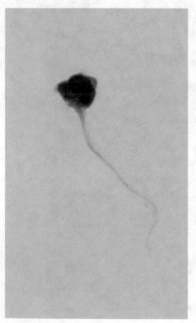

**Fig. 49**  Triple head
*May-Grünwald-Giemsa1000×*

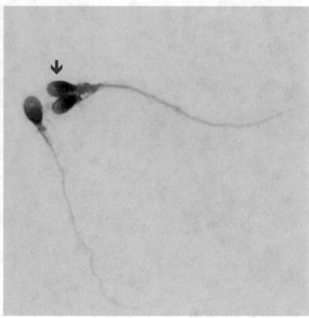

**Fig. 50**  ➔ Double head
*May-Grünwald-Giemsa1000×*

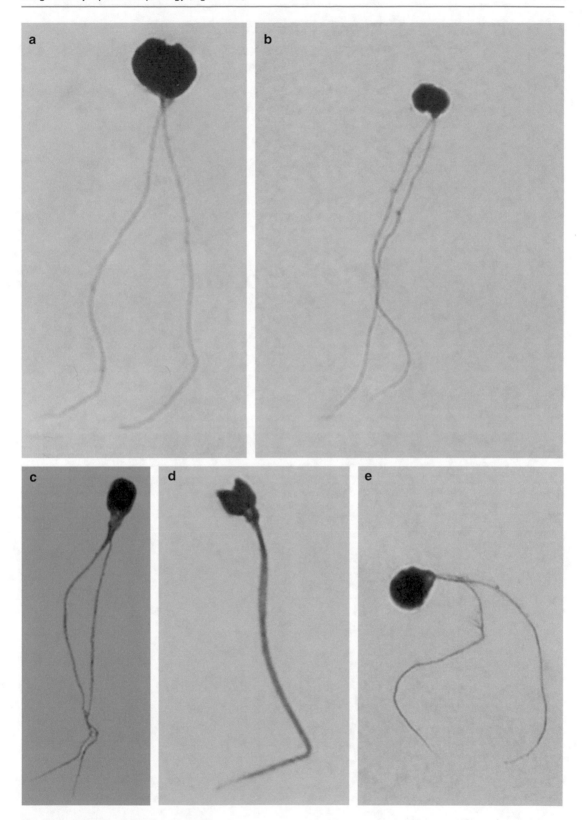

**Fig. 51  a, b, c, d, e** Double heads, double tails
*May-Grünwald-Giemsa1000×*

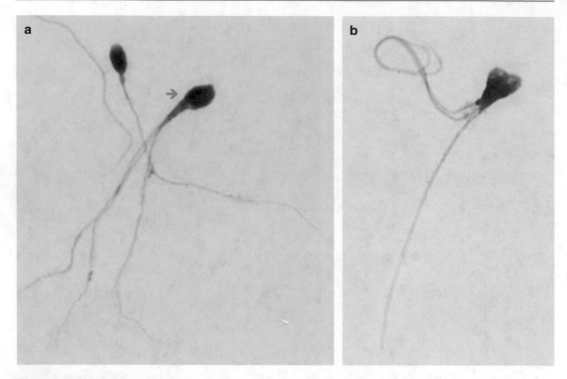

**Fig. 52   a, b** ➡ Double heads with triple tail
*May-Grünwald-Giemsa1000×*

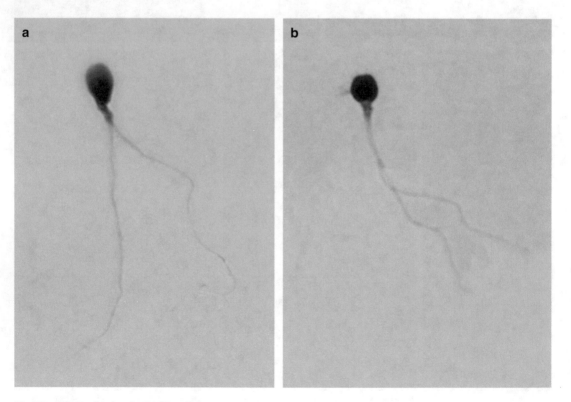

**Fig. 53   a, b** Double heads, double tails
*May-Grünwald-Giemsa1000×*

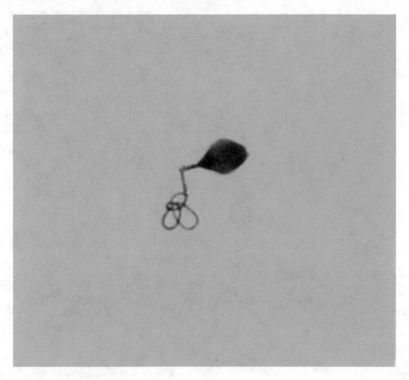

**Fig. 54** Decondensed head
*May-Grünwald-Giemsa1000×*

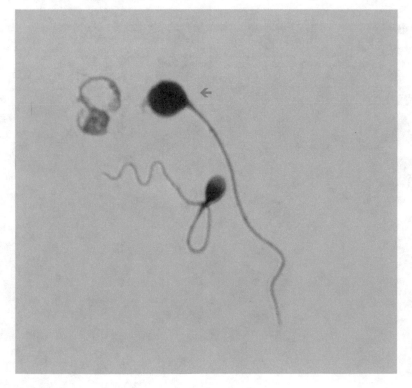

**Fig. 55** → Decondensed head
*May-Grünwald-Giemsa1000×*

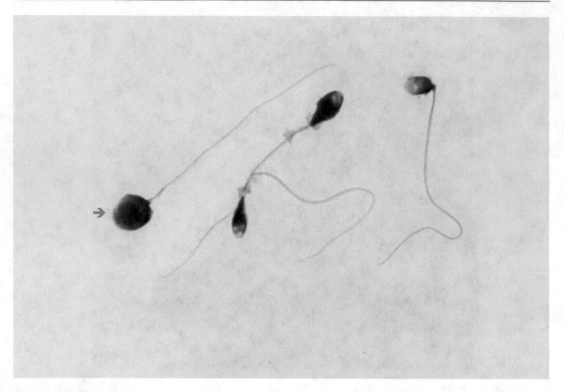

**Fig. 56** ➜ Decondensed head
*May-Grünwald-Giemsa1000×*

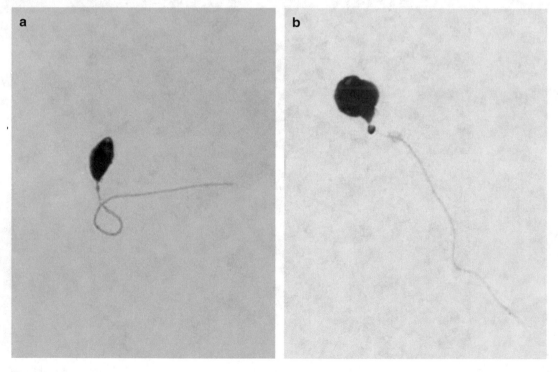

**Fig. 57   a, b** Decondensed heads
*May-Grünwald-Giemsa1000×*

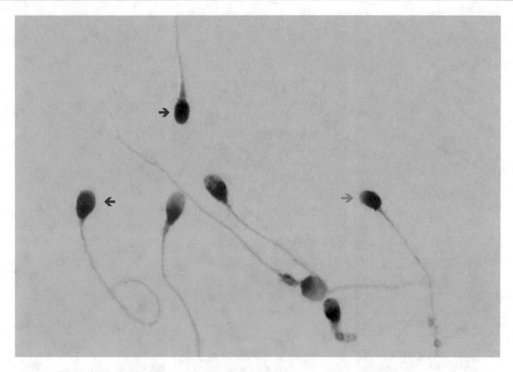

**Fig. 58** ➔ Small acrosomes, ➔ Asymmetrical acrosome
*May-Grünwald-Giemsa1000x*

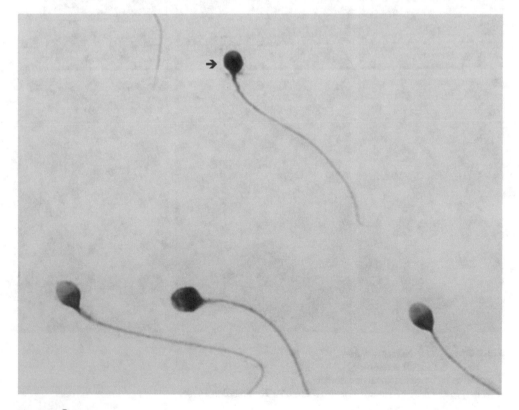

**Fig. 59** ➔ Small acrosome
*May-Grünwald-Giemsa1000x*

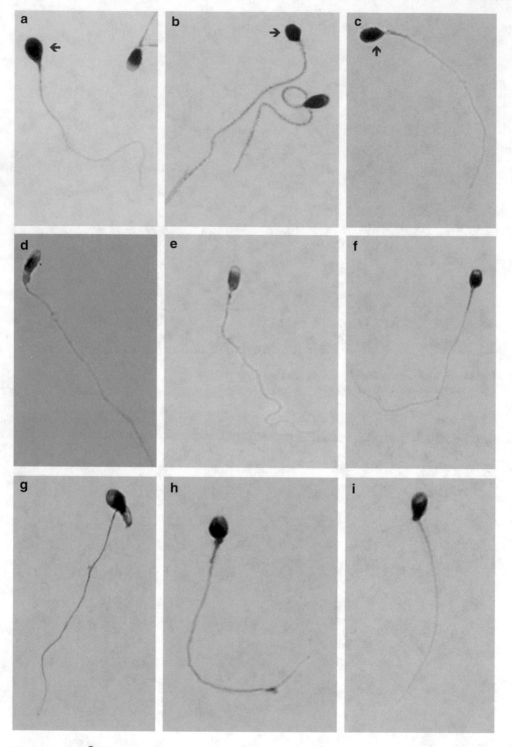

**Fig. 60**  **a, b, c** ➜ No acrosomes
             **d, e, f** Small acrosomes
             **g, h, i** Asymmetrical acrosomes
*a, b, c, f, g, h, i May-Grünwald-Giemsa1000x, d, e Papanicolau 1000×*

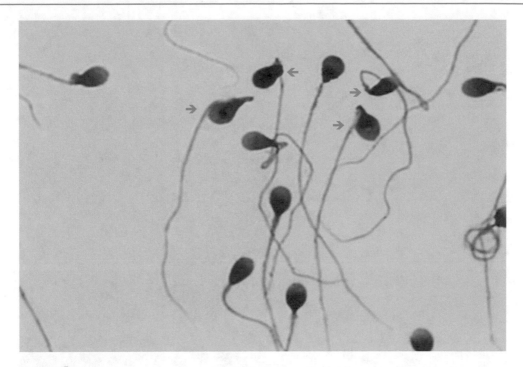

**Fig. 61** ➜ Bent necks
*May-Grünwald-Giemsa1000×*

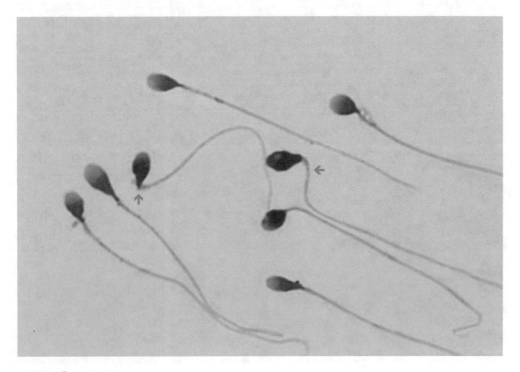

**Fig. 62** ➜ Bent necks
*May-Grünwald-Giemsa1000×*

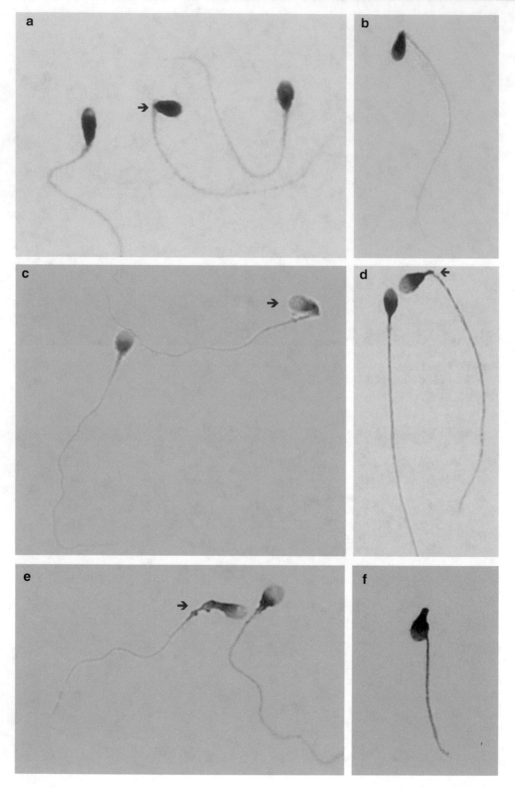

**Fig. 63**   a, b, c, d, e, f ➡ Bent necks
*a, b, d, f May-Grünwald-Giemsa1000×, c, e Papanicolau 1000×*

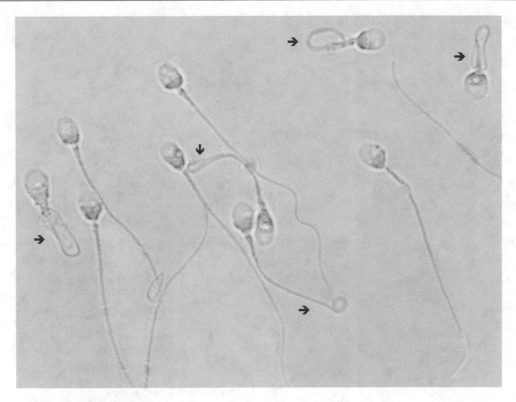

**Fig. 64** ➜ Looped tails
*Unstained 1000×*

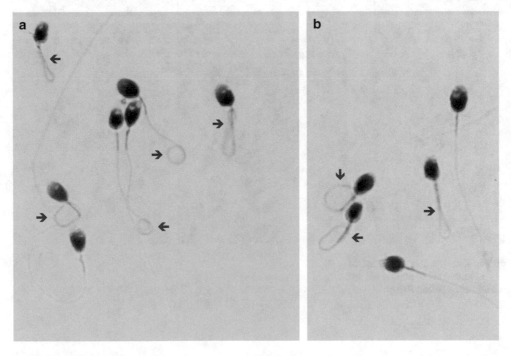

**Fig. 65   a, b** ➜ Looped tails
*Diff Quik 1000×*

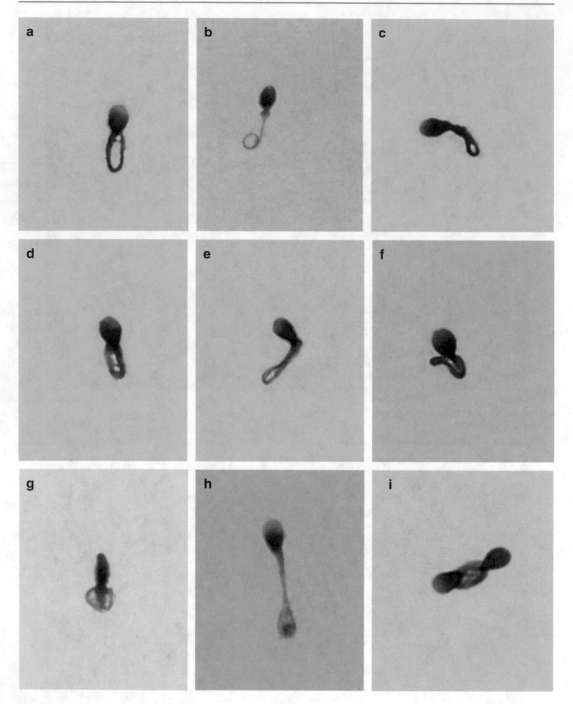

**Fig. 66**   **a**, **b**, **c**, **d**, **e**, **f**, **g**, **h** Looped tails
       **i** Double head, double tail and looped tail
*May-Grünwald-Giemsa1000×*

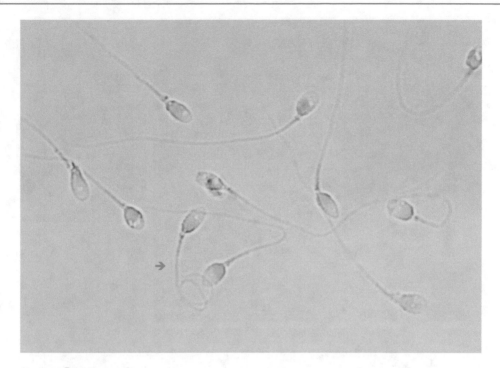

**Fig. 67** ➔ Coiled tail
*Unstained 1000×*

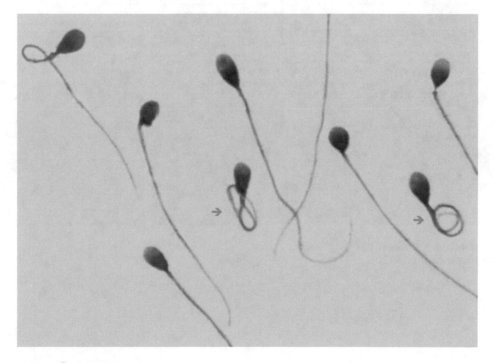

**Fig. 68** ➔ Coiled tails
*May-Grünwald-Giemsa1000×*

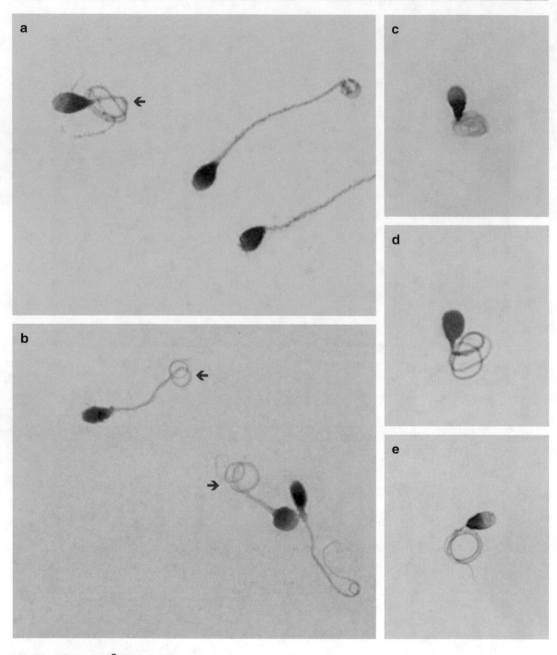

**Fig. 69** a, b, c, d, e ➔ Coiled tails
*May-Grünwald-Giemsa1000×*

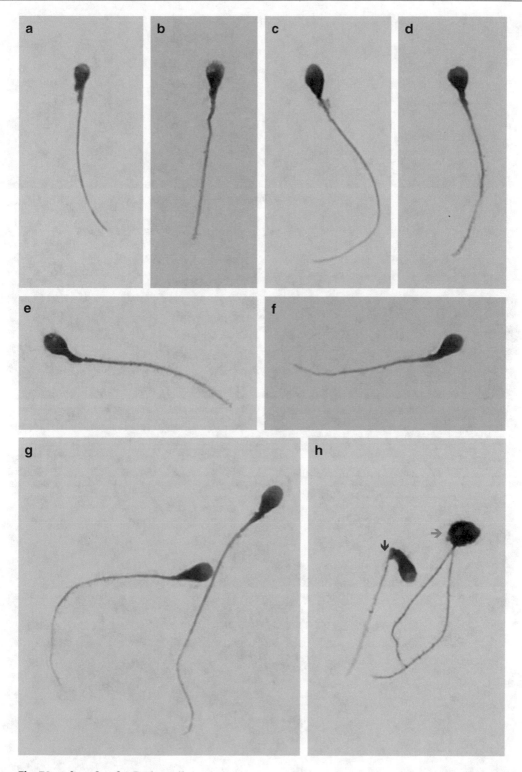

**Fig. 70**   **a, b, c, d, e, f, g** Broken tails
                **h ➜** Broken tail, ➜ Double head, Double tail and broken tails
*May-Grünwald-Giemsa1000×*

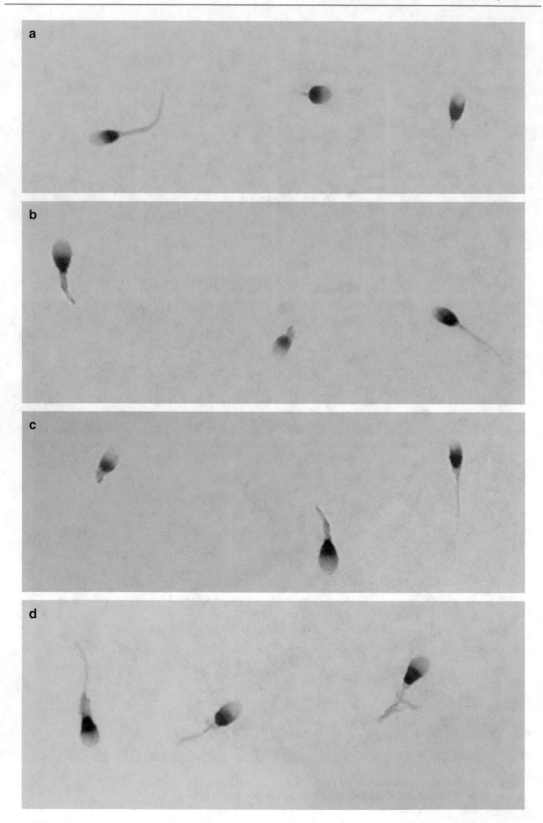

**Fig. 71  a**, **b**, **c**, **d** Broken tails and short tails
*May-Grünwald-Giemsa1000×*

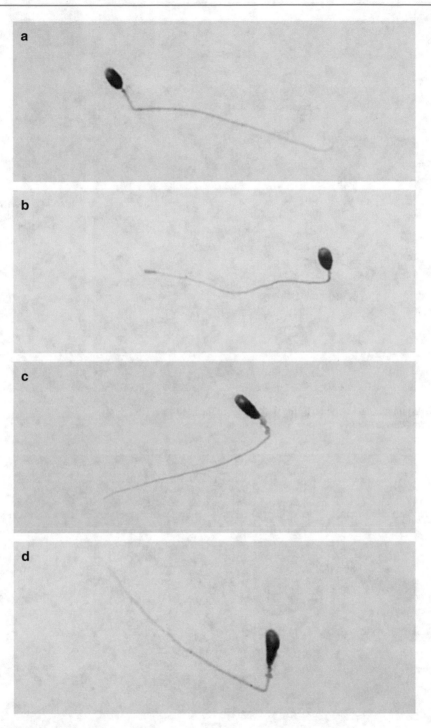

**Fig. 72** **a**, **b**, **c**, **d** Bent tails
*May-Grünwald-Giemsa1000×*

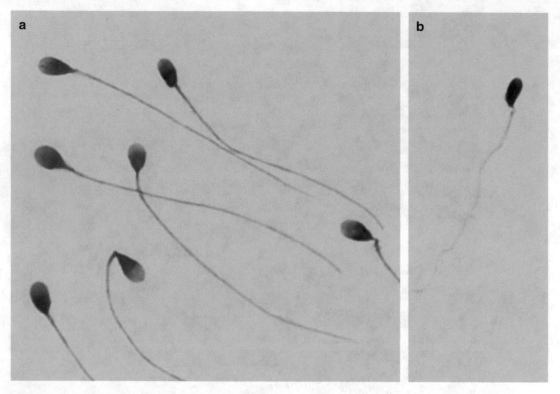

**Fig. 73   a, b** Asymmetrical insertions of the midpiece into the head
*May-Grünwald-Giemsa 1000×*

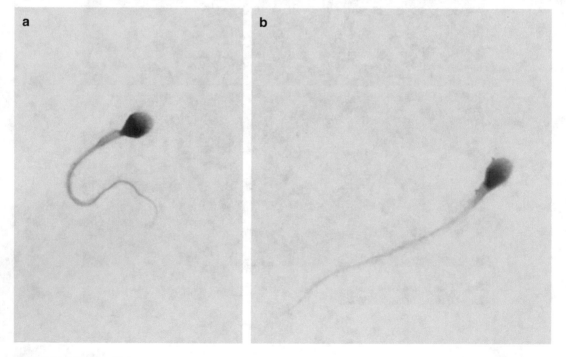

**Fig. 74   a, b** Thick midpieces
*May-Grünwald-Giemsa 1000×*

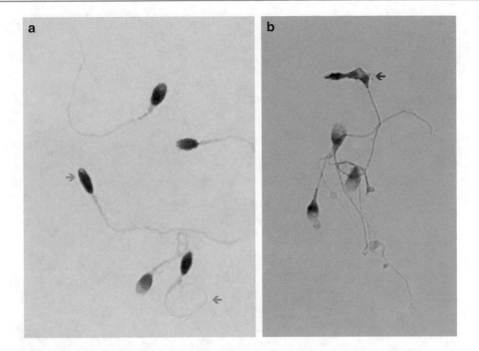

**Fig. 75  a ➔** Tapered head and small and asymmetrical acrosome
           ➔ Tapered head and small acrosome and coiled tail
*May-Grünwald-Giemsa1000×*
       **b ➔** Tapered head without acrosome, bent neck and excess residual cytoplasm
*Papanicolau 1000×*

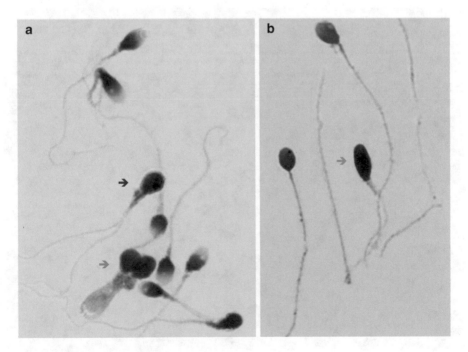

**Fig. 76  a ➔** Round head with double tail
           ➔ Double head, double tail and looped tail
       **b ➔** Large head without acrosome
*May-Grünwald-Giemsa1000×*

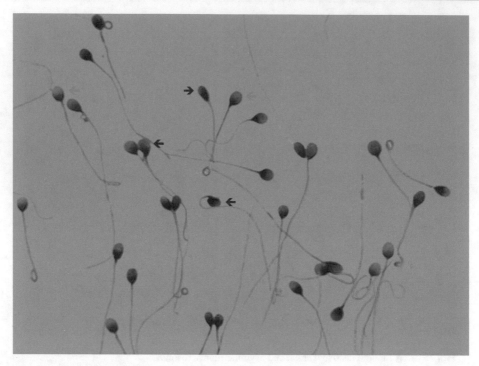

**Fig. 77** ➔ Normal heads,
➔ Amorphous heads
*May-Grünwald-Giemsa1000×*

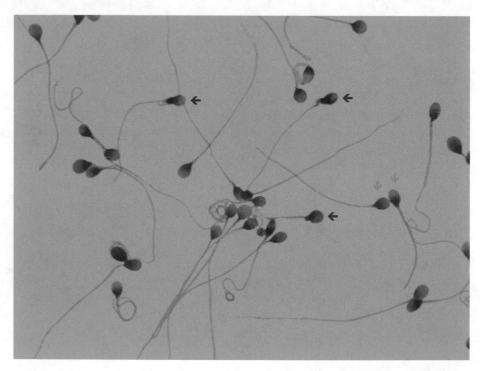

**Fig. 78** ➔ Normal heads,
➔ Amorphous heads
*May-Grünwald-Giemsa1000×*

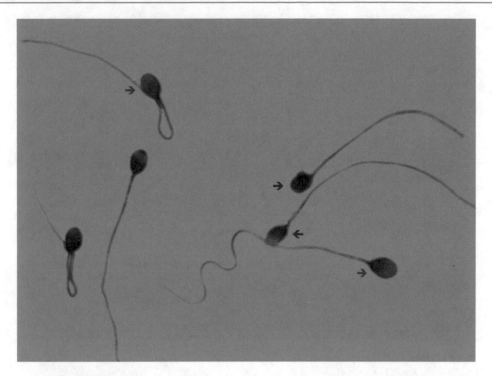

**Fig. 79**  ➔ Normal heads,
➔ Amorphous heads
*May-Grünwald-Giemsa1000×*

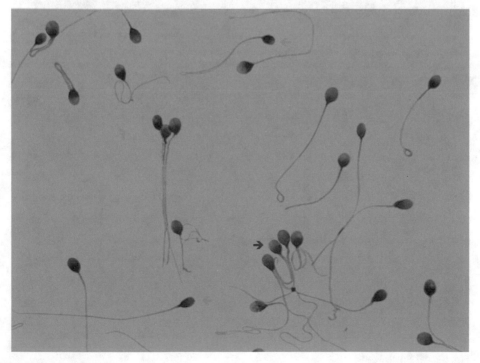

**Fig. 80**  ➔ Small heads,
➔ Normal heads
*May-Grünwald-Giemsa1000×*

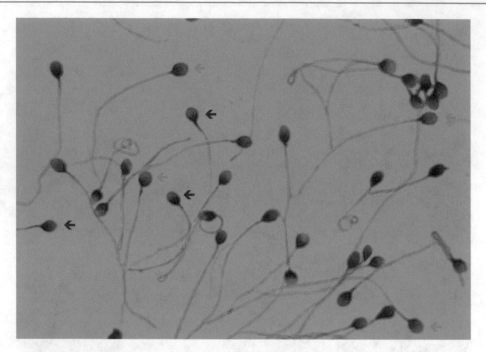

**Fig. 81** ➜ Normal heads,
➜ Small heads
*May-Grünwald-Giemsa1000×*

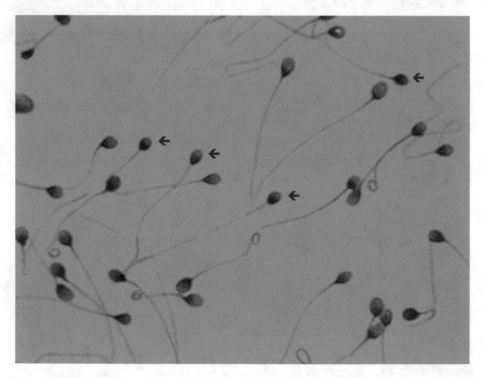

**Fig. 82** ➜ Small heads
*May-Grünwald-Giemsa1000×*

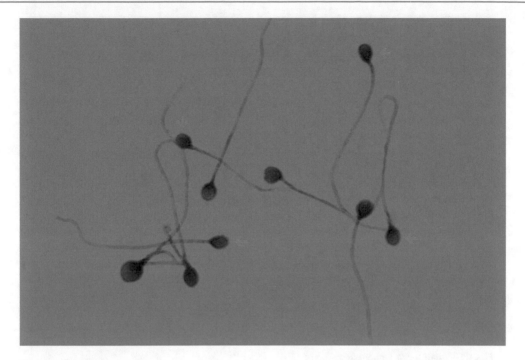

**Fig. 83** → Small heads
*May-Grünwald-Giemsa1000×*

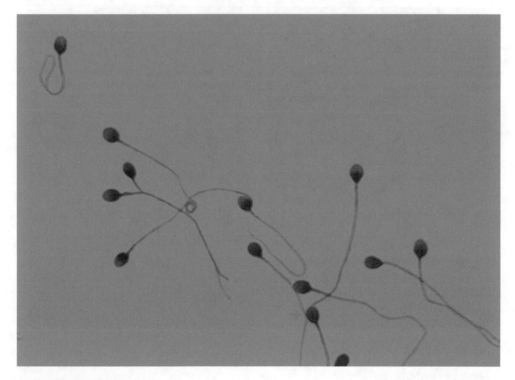

**Fig. 84** → Small heads
*May-Grünwald-Giemsa1000×*

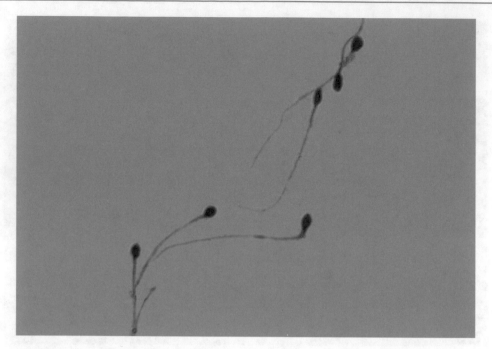

**Fig. 85** Small heads without acrosome
*May-Grünwald-Giemsa1000×*

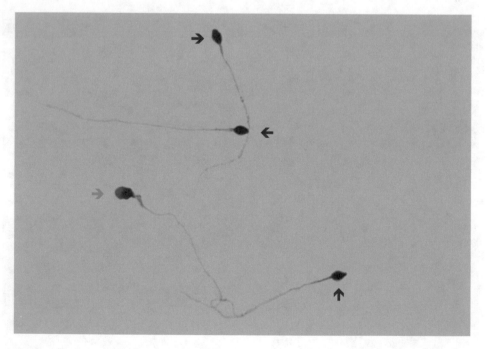

**Fig. 86** ➜ Small heads without acrosome,
            ➜ Amorphous head
*May-Grünwald-Giemsa1000×*

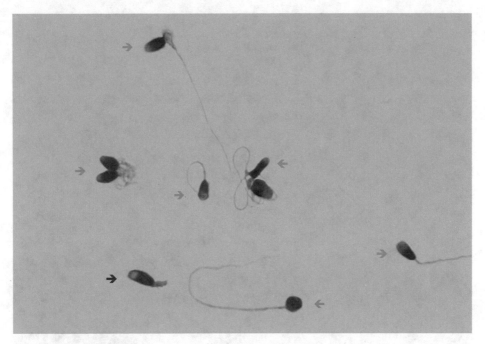

**Fig. 87** ➔ Amorphous heads,                    ➔ Tapered head,
      ➔ Amorphous head and short tail,    ➔ Round head
*May-Grünwald-Giemsa1000×*

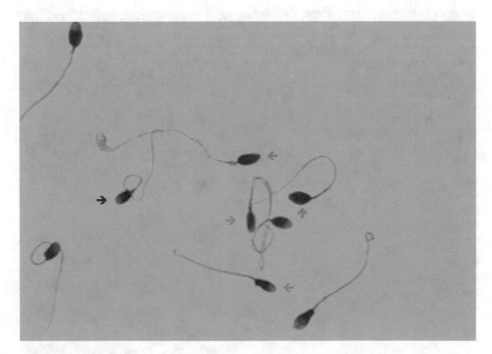

**Fig. 88** ➔ Amorphous heads with no acrosome,    ➔ Small head
      ➔ Tapered heads and small acrosome
*May-Grünwald-Giemsa1000×*

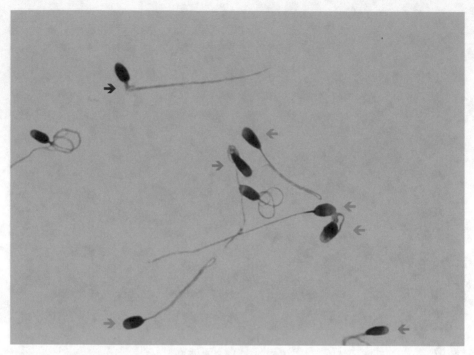

**Fig. 89**  ➔ Tapered heads,        ➔ Amorphous heads,
              ➔ Bent and broken tail
*May-Grünwald-Giemsa1000×*

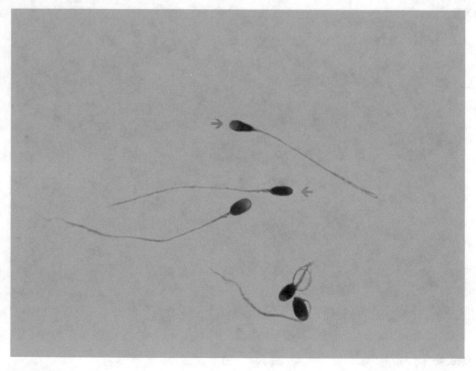

**Fig. 90**  ➔ Pyriform head,
              ➔ Small head and broken tail
*May-Grünwald-Giemsa1000×*

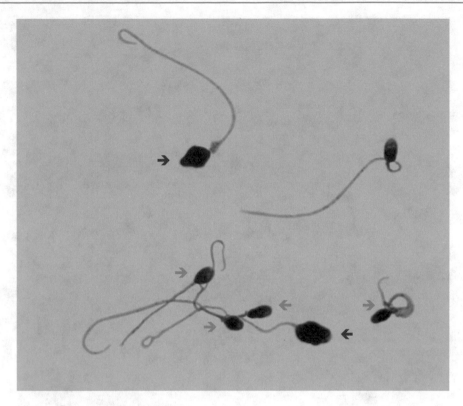

**Fig. 91** ➔ Large heads,
➔ Small heads
*May-Grünwald-Giemsa1000×*

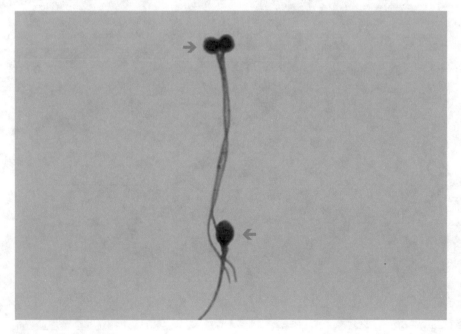

**Fig. 92** ➔ Small head,
➔ Round heads
*May-Grünwald-Giemsa1000×*

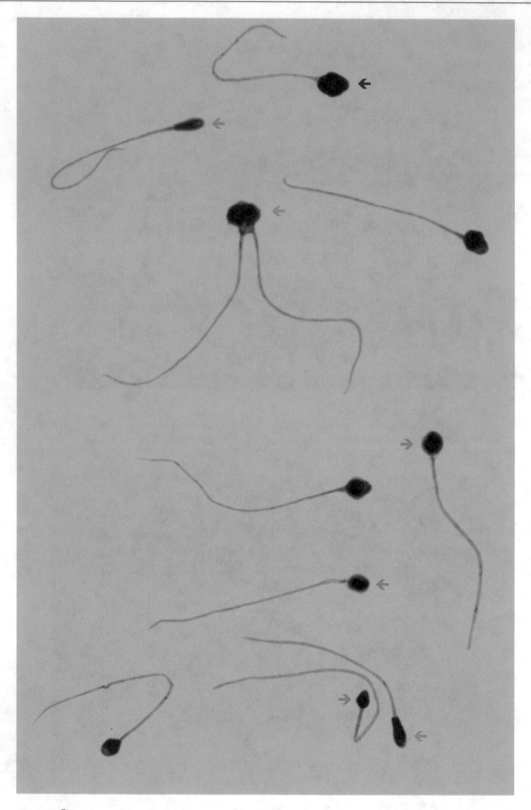

**Fig. 93** ➜ Large head, Double head,          ➜ double tail,
          ➜ Small heads without acrosome     ➜ Tapered heads
*May-Grünwald-Giemsa 1000×*

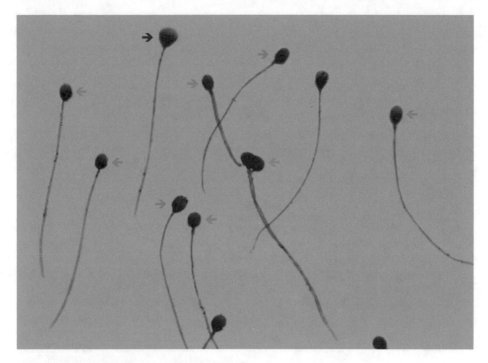

**Fig. 94** ➔ Amorphous heads,   ➔ Small heads,
         ➔ Pyriform head    ➔ Double head, double tail
*May-Grünwald-Giemsa1000×*

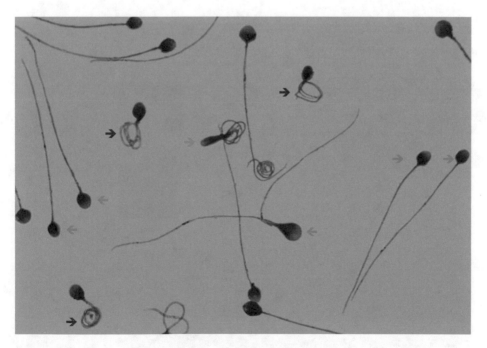

**Fig. 95** ➔ Tapered head and coiled tail,   ➔ small heads
         ➔ Pyriform head with double tail,   ➔ Coiled tails
*May-Grünwald-Giemsa1000×*

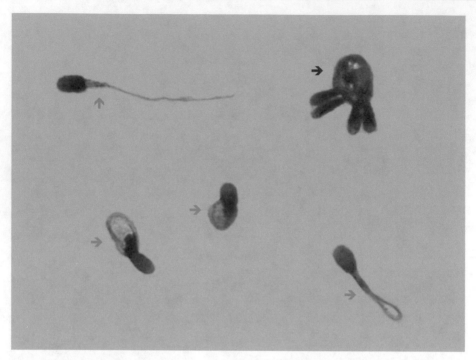

**Fig. 96**  ➜ Looped tails, ➜ Quadruple head, quadruple tail and tapered heads
        ➜ Broken tail
*May-Grünwald-Giemsa1000×*

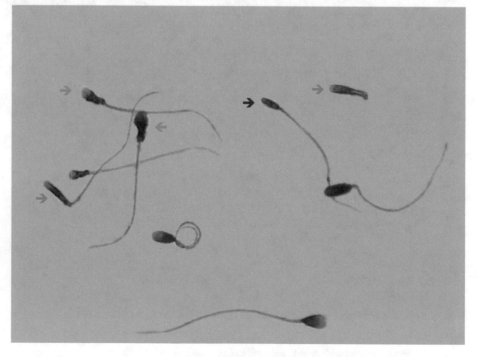

**Fig. 97**  ➜ Tapered head,          ➜ Tapered head and bent neck and broken tail
        ➜ Amorphous heads,        ➜ Tapered head and short tail
*May-Grünwald-Giemsa1000×*

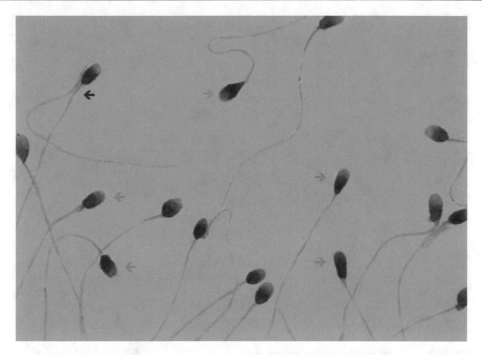

**Fig. 98** ➜ Amorphous heads,   ➜ Tapered heads,
           ➜ Pyriform head,      ➜ Double tail
*May-Grünwald-Giemsa1000×*

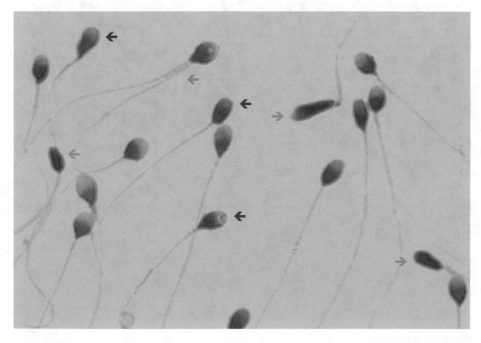

**Fig. 99** ➜ Amorphous heads,   ➜ Tapered heads,
           ➜ Double tail         ➜ Small head without acrosome
*May-Grünwald-Giemsa1000×*

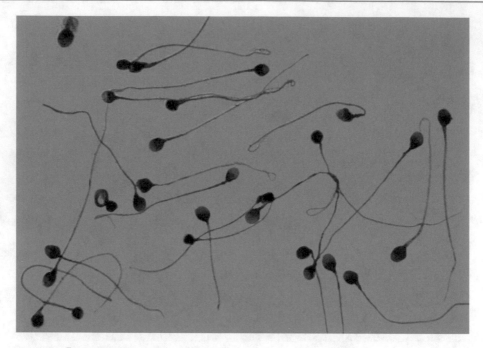

**Fig. 100** ➜ Small heads without acrosome
*May-Grünwald-Giemsa1000×*

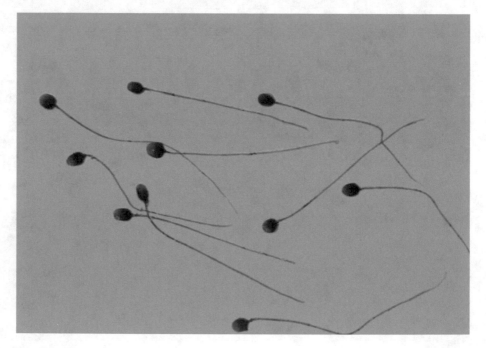

**Fig. 101** Small heads
*May-Grünwald-Giemsa1000×*

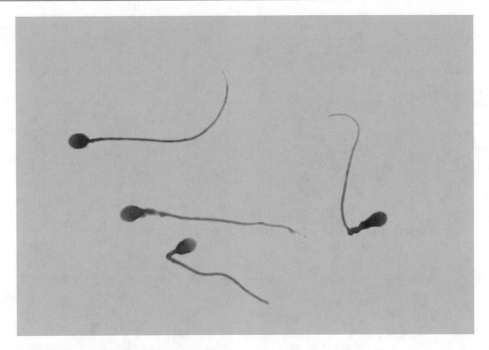

**Fig. 102**  Amorphous heads and broken tails
*May-Grünwald-Giemsa1000×*

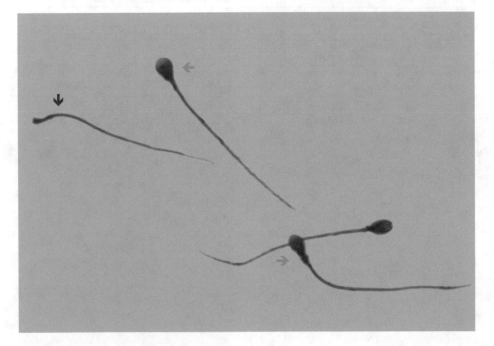

**Fig. 103**  → Pyriform heads and broken tails,
→ Pinhead and broken tail
*May-Grünwald-Giemsa1000×*

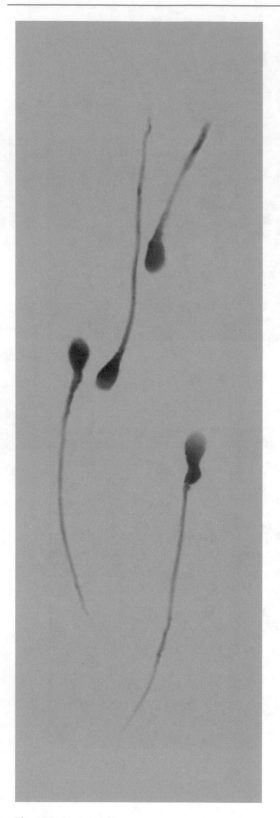

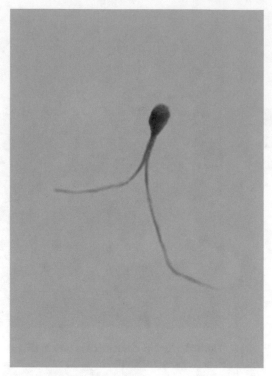

**Fig. 105** Double and broken tail
*May-Grünwald-Giemsa1000×*

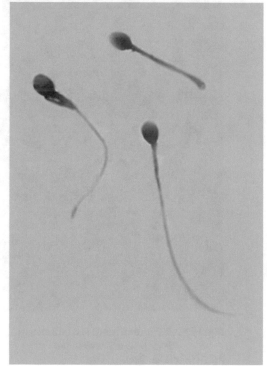

**Fig. 104** Broken tails,
*May-Grünwald-Giemsa1000×*

**Fig. 106** Broken tails
*May-Grünwald-Giemsa1000×*

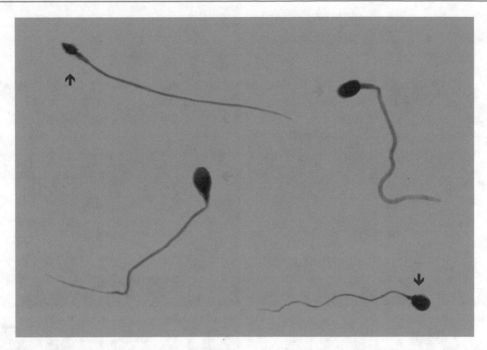

**Fig. 107** ➜ Small heads,
➜ Amorphous heads
*May-Grünwald-Giemsa1000×*

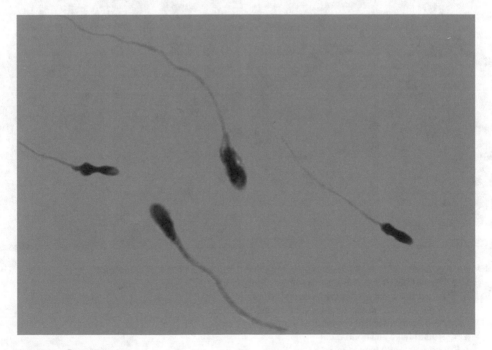

**Fig. 108** ➜ Tapered heads,
➜ Amorphous head
*May-Grünwald-Giemsa1000×*

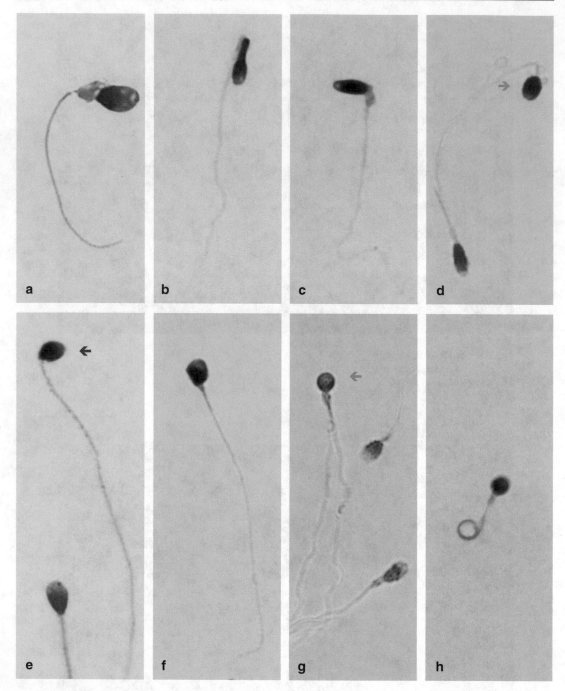

**Fig. 109**  **a** Large head and vacuolated acrosome, broken tail and excess residual cytoplasm
  **b, c** Tapered heads and small acrosome and bent neck
  **d** ➜ Small head and small acrosome and bent tail
  **e** ➜ Amorphous head and small acrosome and bent neck
  **f** Amorphous head and asymmetrical acrosome
  **g** ➜ Round head and double tail
  **h** Round head with looped tail
*a, b, c, d, e, f, h May-Grünwald-Giemsa1000×, g Papanicolau 1000×*

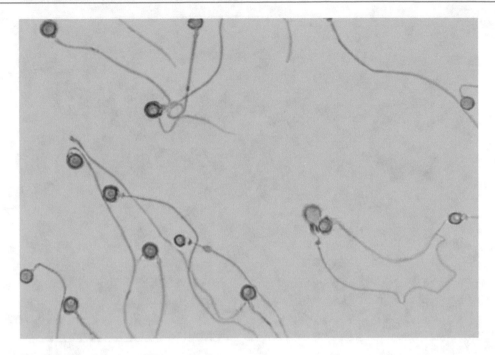

**Fig. 110**   Round heads
*Unstained 1000×*

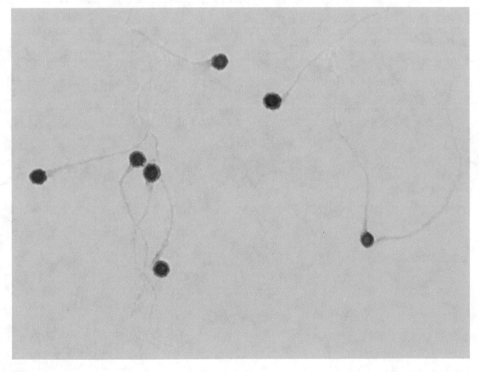

**Fig. 111**   Round heads
*May-Grünwald-Giemsa1000×*

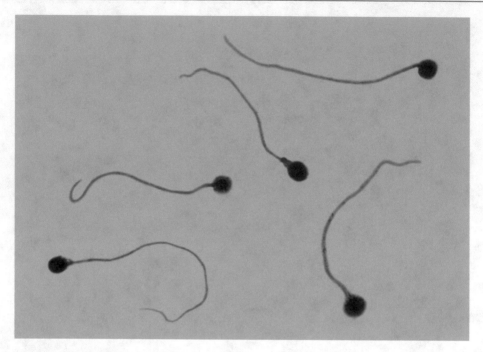

**Fig. 112**  Round heads
*May-Grünwald-Giemsa1000×*

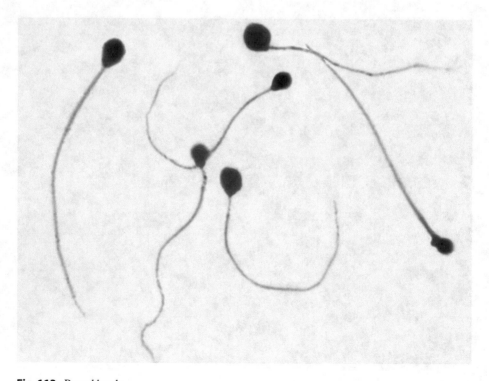

**Fig. 113**  Round heads
*May-Grünwald-Giemsa1000×*

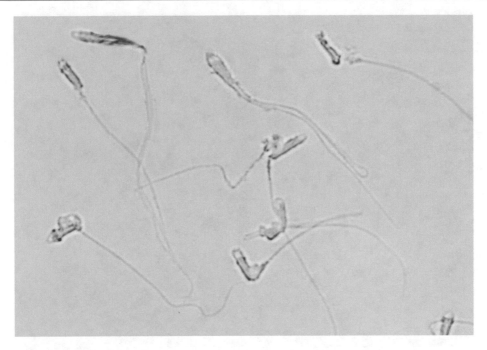

**Fig. 114** Tapered heads
*Unstained 1000×*

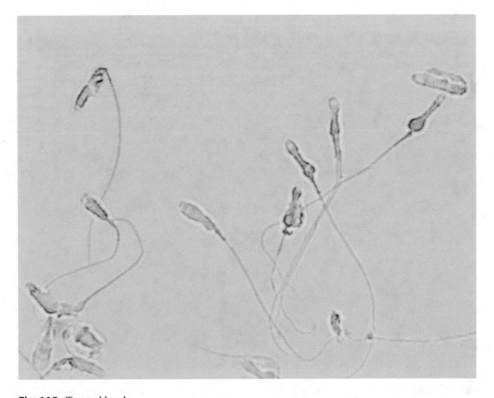

**Fig. 115** Tapered heads
*Unstained 1000×*

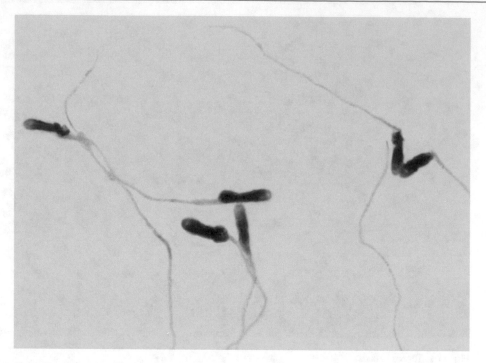

**Fig. 116** Tapered heads
*May-Grünwald-Giemsa1000×*

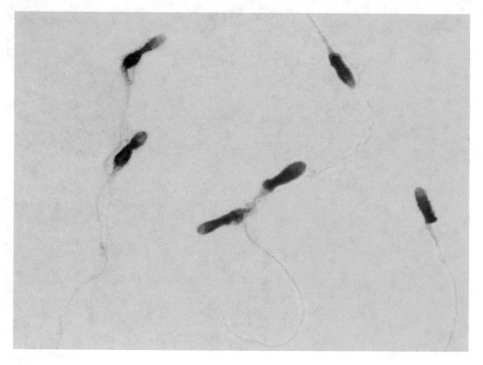

**Fig. 117** Tapered heads
*May-Grünwald-Giemsa1000×*

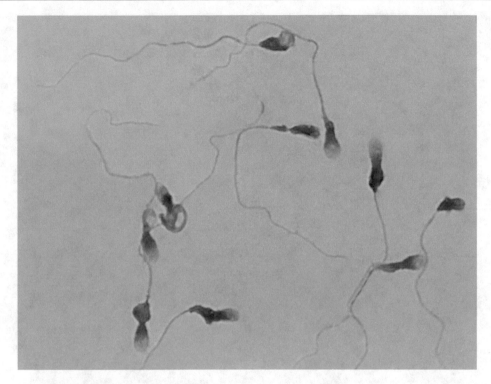

**Fig. 118** Excess residual cytoplasm
*Papanicolau 1000×*

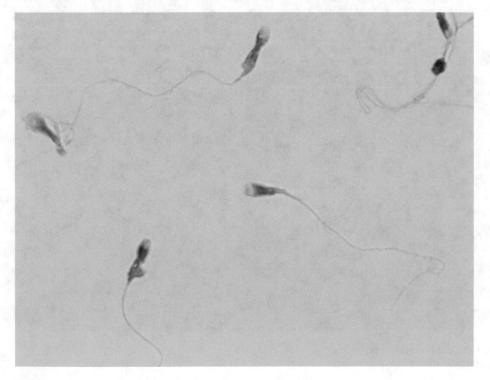

**Fig. 119** Excess residual cytoplasm
*Papanicolau 1000×*

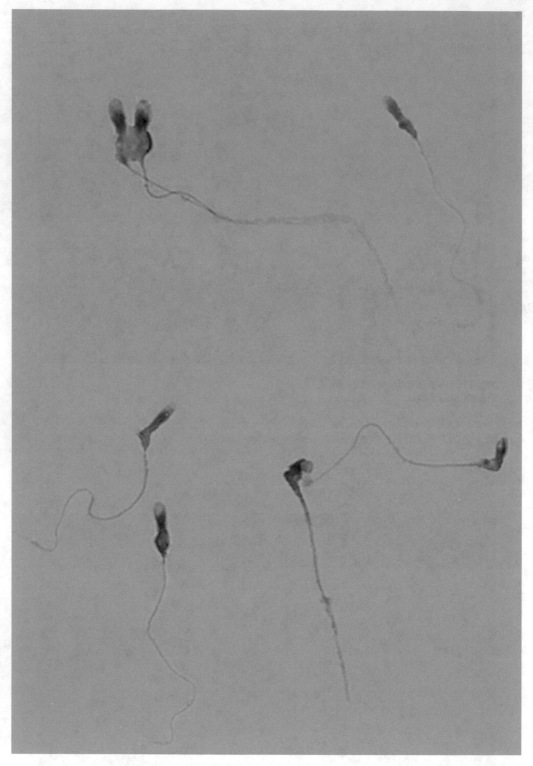

**Fig. 120**  Excess residual cytoplasm
*Papanicolau 1000×*

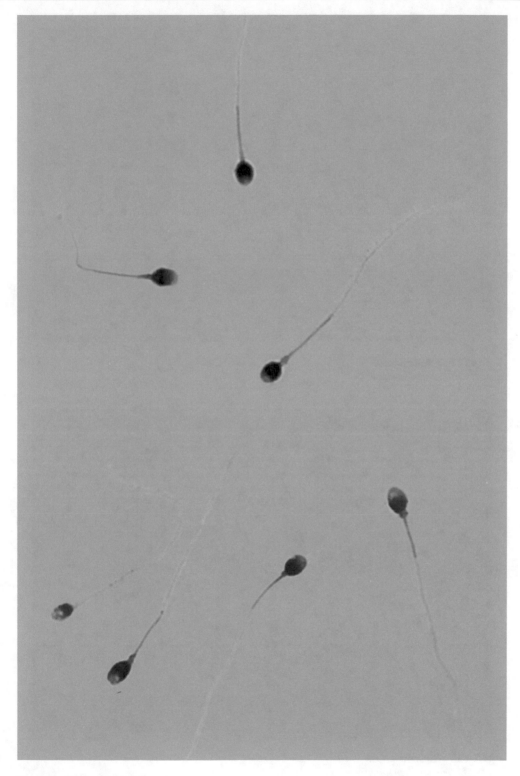

**Fig. 121**  Thick midpieces
*May-Grünwald-Giemsa1000×*

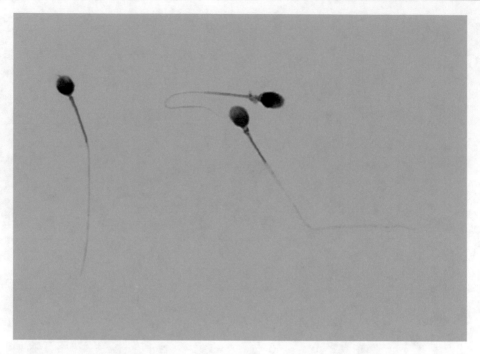

**Fig. 122** Thick midpieces
*May-Grünwald-Giemsa1000×*

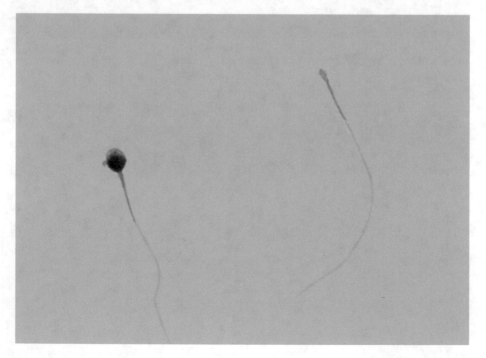

**Fig. 123** Thick midpieces
*May-Grünwald-Giemsa1000×*

# Image Gallery: Non-Sperm Cellular Components (Figs. 124–150)

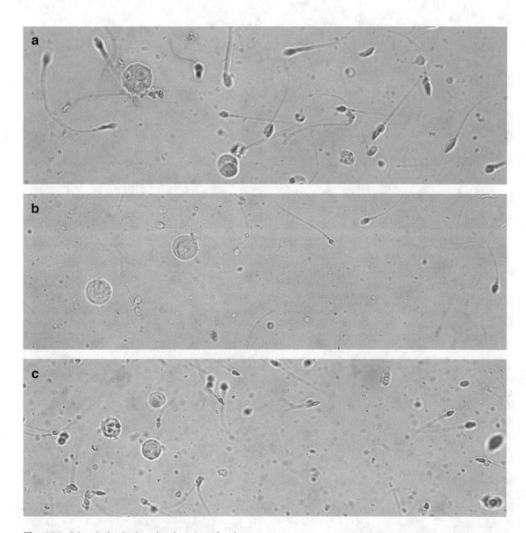

**Fig. 124** Morphological evaluation, unstained
**a, b, c** Spermatozoa and germ cells
*Unstained 400×*

© Springer Nature Switzerland AG 2020
D. Paoli et al., *Atlas of Human Semen Examination*, Trends in Andrology and Sexual Medicine,
https://doi.org/10.1007/978-3-030-39998-6_4

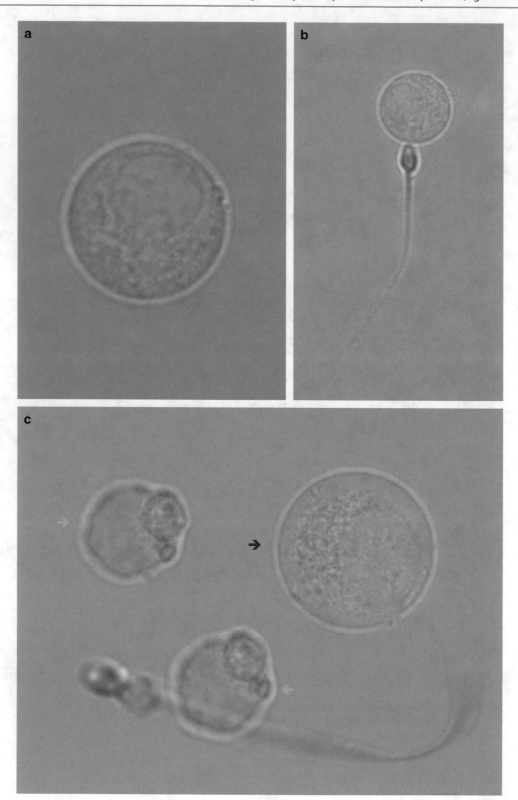

**Fig. 125**  Morphological evaluation, unstained
   **a, b** Primary spermatocyte
   **c** ➜ Primary spermatocyte, ➜ Spermatids
*Unstained 1000×*

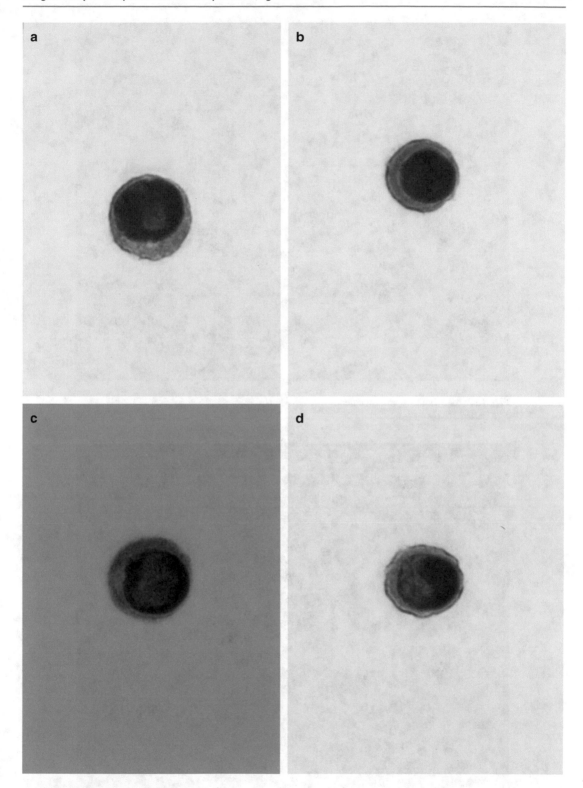

**Fig. 126**  **a**, **b**, **c**, **d** Spermatogonia
*May-Grünwald-Giemsa 1000×*

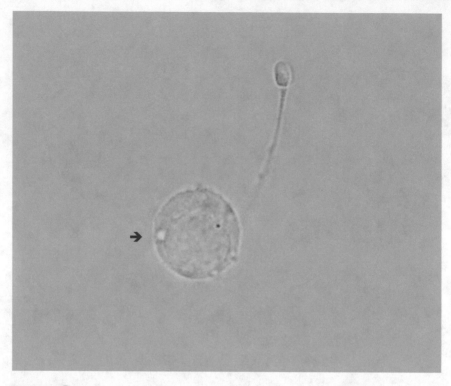

**Fig. 127** ➜ Primary spermatocyte
*Unstained 1000×*

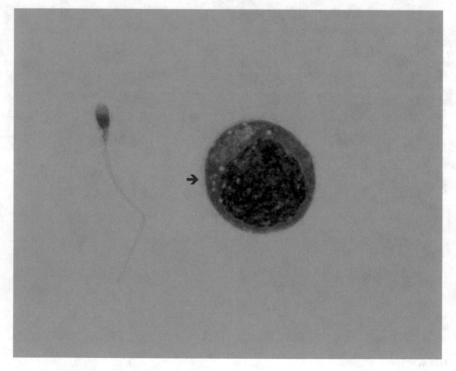

**Fig. 128** ➜ Primary spermatocyte
*May-Grünwald-Giemsa 1000×*

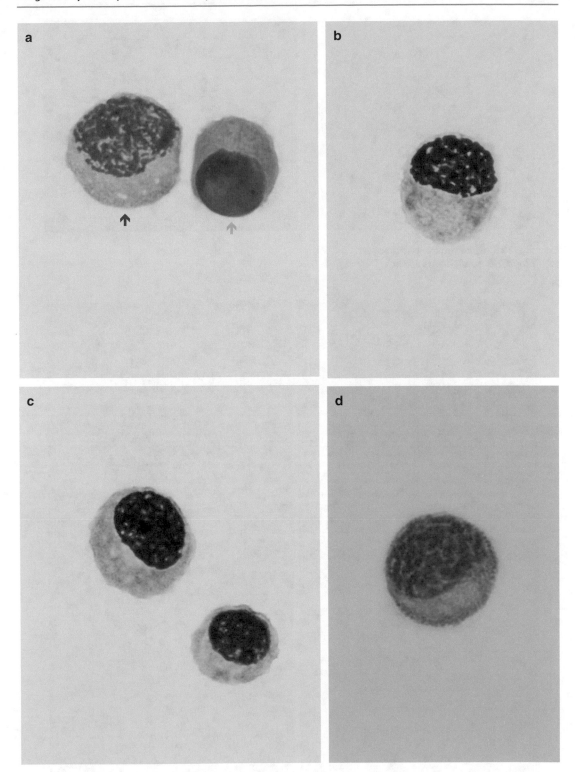

**Fig. 129**  a ➜ Primary spermatocyte, ➜ Spermatogonium
      **b, c, d** Primary spermatocytes
*May-Grünwald-Giemsa 1000×*

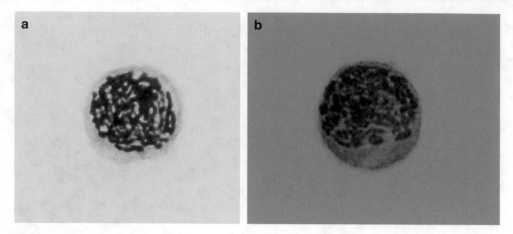

**Fig. 130  a, b** Primary spermatocytes
*May-Grünwald-Giemsa 1000×*

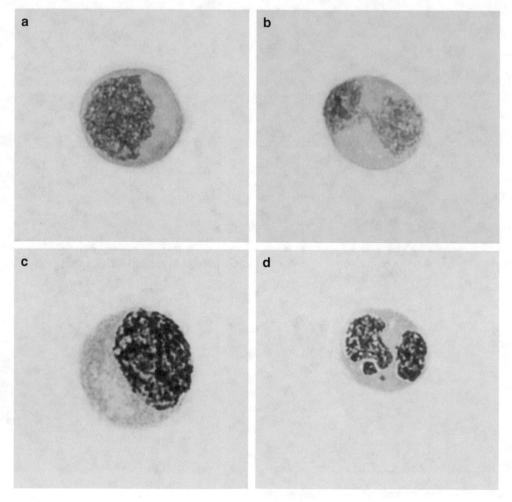

**Fig. 131  a, c** Primary spermatocytes
         **b, d** Primary spermatocytes during meiotic division
*May-Grünwald-Giemsa 1000×*

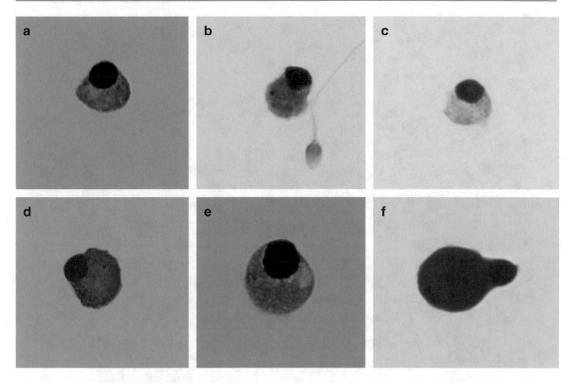

**Fig. 132**  a, b, c, d, e, f Spermatids
*May-Grünwald-Giemsa 1000×*

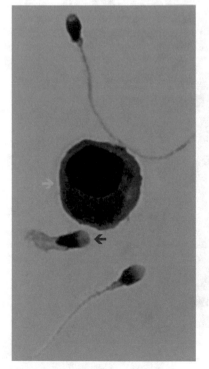

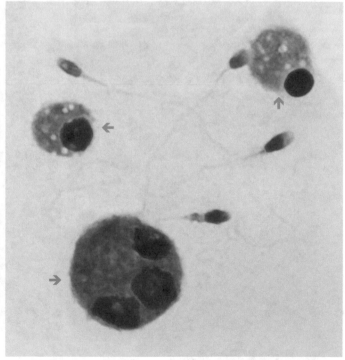

**Fig. 133**  ➜ Round spermatid
➜ Elongated spermatid
*May-Grünwald-Giemsa 1000×*

**Fig. 134**  ➜ Spermatids
➜ Trinuclear cell
*May-Grünwald-Giemsa 1000×*

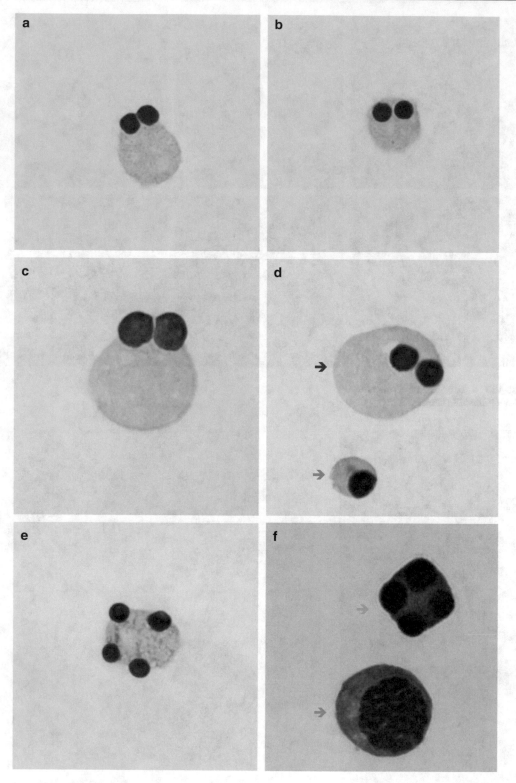

**Fig. 135**  **a, b, c** Binuclear cells
**d** ➜ Binuclear cell, ➜ Spermatid
**e** Tetranuclear cell
**f** ➜ Tetranuclear cell, ➜ Primary spermatocyte
*May-Grünwald-Giemsa 1000×*

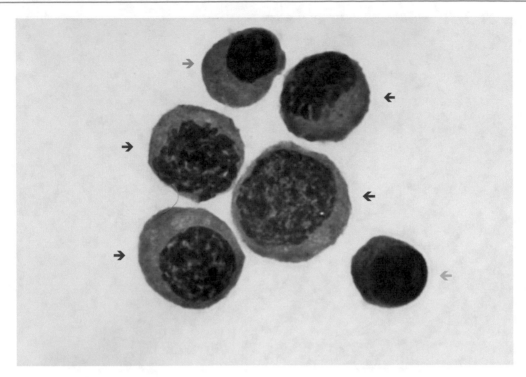

**Fig. 136** ➜ Primary spermatocytes
      ➜ Secondary spermatocyte
      ➜ Spermatid
*May-Grünwald-Giemsa 1000×*

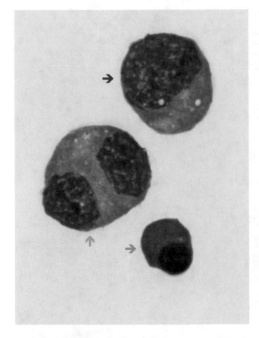

**Fig. 137** ➜ Primary spermatocyte
      ➜ Binuclear cell
      ➜ Spermatid
*May-Grünwald-Giemsa 1000×*

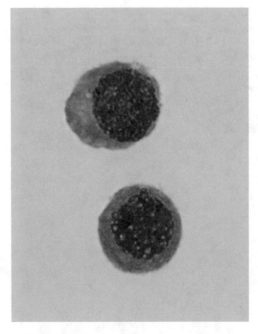

**Fig. 138** Primary spermatocytes
*May-Grünwald-Giemsa 1000×*

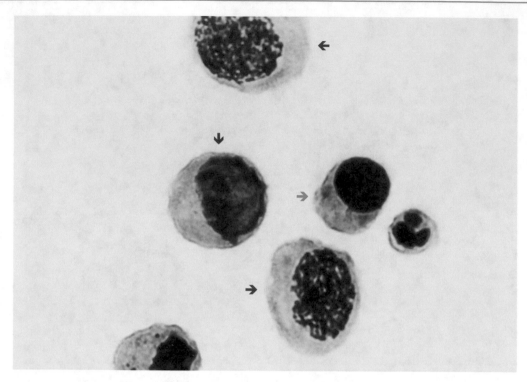

**Fig. 139** ➜ Primary spermatocytes
            ➜ Spermatid
*May-Grünwald-Giemsa 1000×*

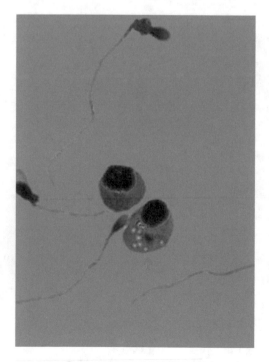

**Fig. 140** ➜ Spermatid
*May-Grünwald-Giemsa 1000×*

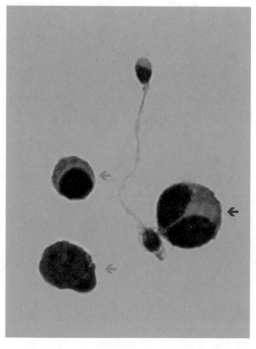

**Fig. 141** ➜ Binuclear primary spermatocyte
            ➜ Spermatids
*May-Grünwald-Giemsa 1000×*

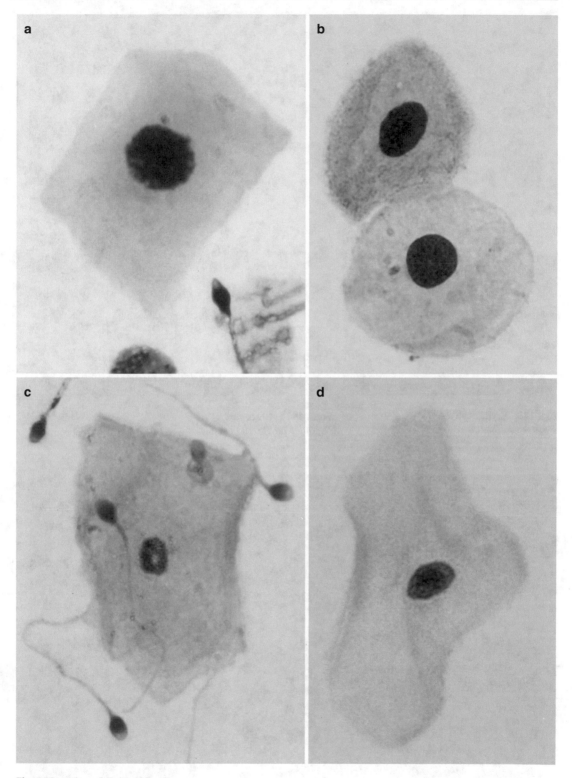

**Fig. 142  a, b, c, d** Epithelial cells
*May-Grünwald-Giemsa 1000×*

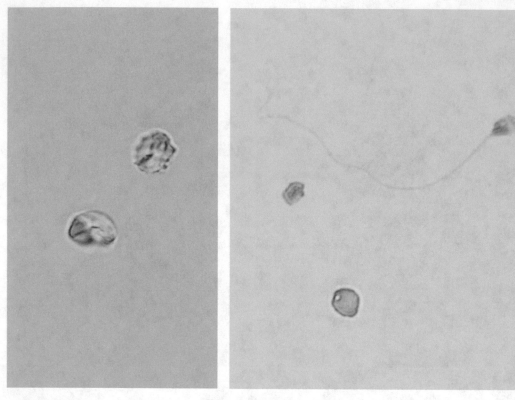

**Fig. 143** Erythrocytes
*Unstained 1000x*

**Fig. 144** Erythrocytes
*Papanicolau 1000×*

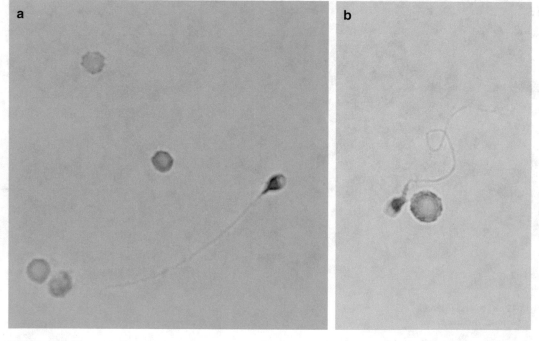

**Fig. 145  a, b** Erythrocytes
*Papanicolau 1000×*

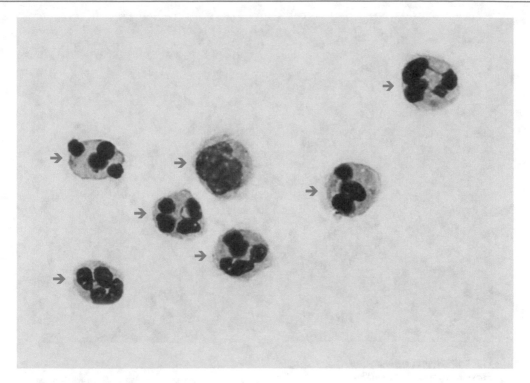

**Fig. 146** ➜ Polymorphonuclear cells
        ➜ Primary spermatocyte
*May-Grünwald-Giemsa 1000×*

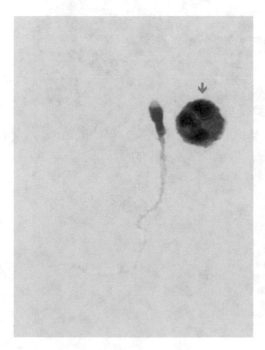

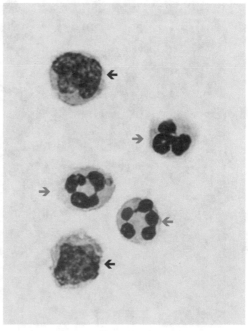

**Fig. 147** ➜ Polymorphonuclear cell
*May-Grünwald-Giemsa 1000×*

**Fig. 148** ➜ Polymorphonuclear cells
        ➜ Primary spermatocytes
*May-Grünwald-Giemsa 1000×*

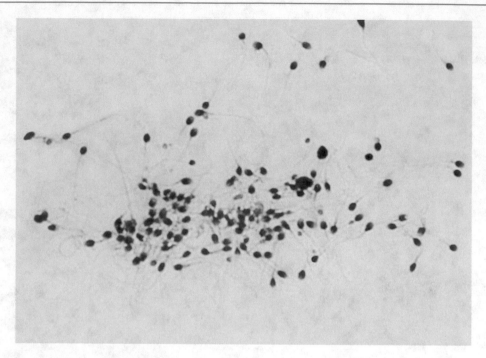

**Fig. 149**  Sperm agglutination
*May-Grünwald-Giemsa 400×*

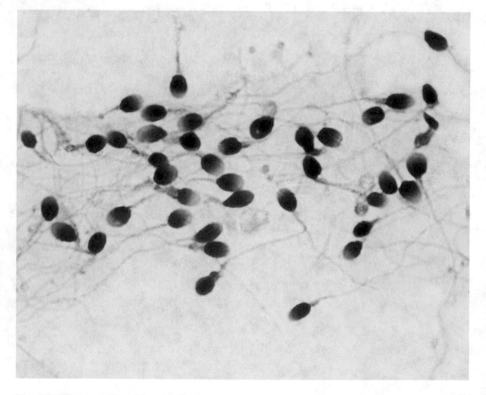

**Fig. 150**  Sperm agglutination
*May-Grünwald-Giemsa 1000×*

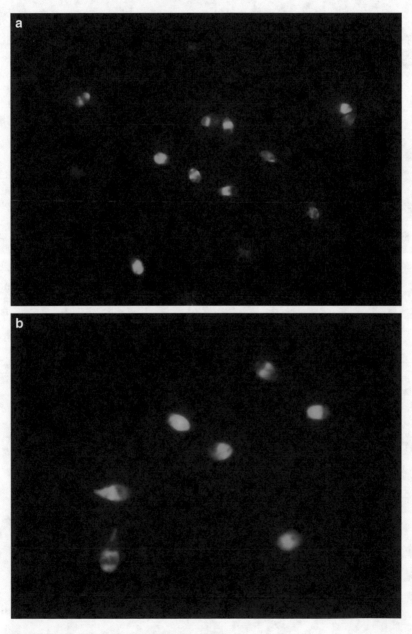

**Fig. 151** **a**, **b** Sperm Fluorescent heads with fragmented DNA
*Tunel assay, fluorescence microscope 1000x*

© Springer Nature Switzerland AG 2020

D. Paoli et al., *Atlas of Human Semen Examination*, Trends in Andrology and Sexual Medicine,
https://doi.org/10.1007/978-3-030-39998-6_5

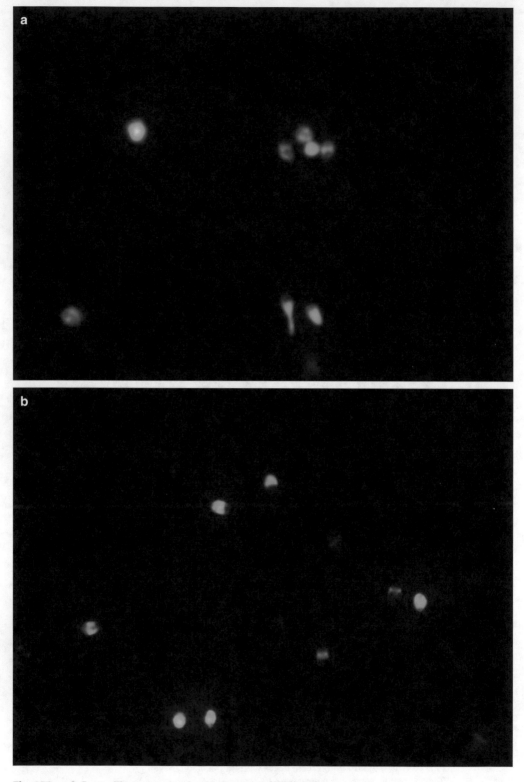

**Fig. 152   a, b** Sperm Fluorescent heads with fragmented DNA
*Tunel assay, fluorescence microscope 1000x*

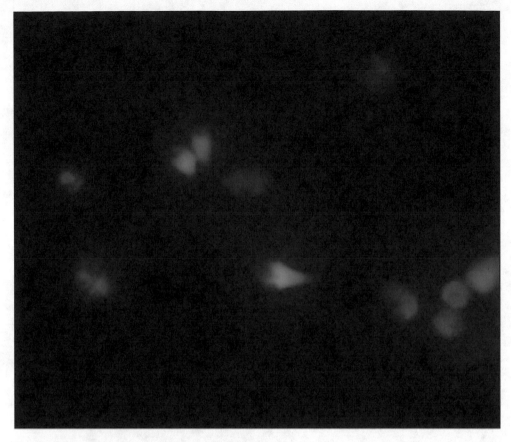

**Fig. 153** Sperm Fluorescent heads with fragmented DNA
*Tunel assay, fluorescence microscope 1000x*

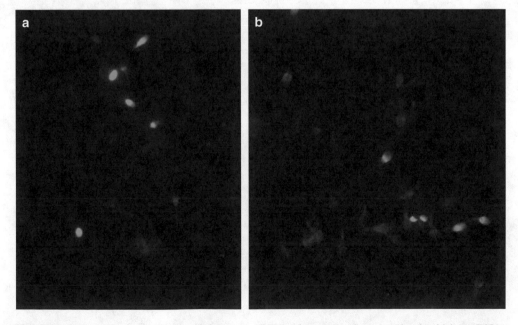

**Fig. 154  a, b** Sperm Fluorescent heads with fragmented DNA and sperm non-fluorescent heads with intact DNA
*Tunel assay, fluorescence microscope 500x*

# Image Gallery: Morphological Evaluation of Sperm Heads with Fragmented DNA, Using Both Transmitted (Bright Field) and Reflected (Dark Field) Light; Every Picture is Shown in Three Different Light Condition

*(Tunel assay, fluorescence microscope - 1000x)*
(Figs. 155–174)

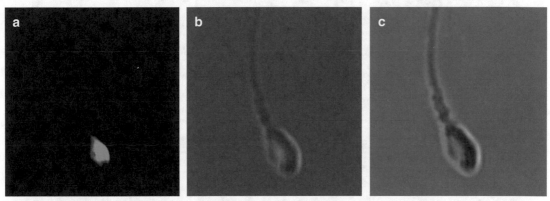

**Fig. 155  a, b** Spermatozoon with fragmented DNA (fluorescent head)
**c** Amorphous head

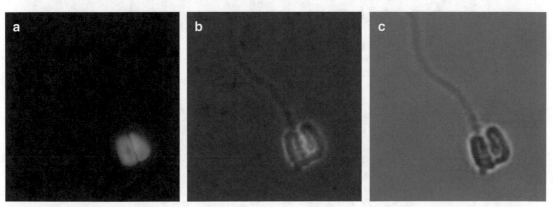

**Fig. 156  a** Two heads with fragmented DNA (fluorescent)
**b** Double head (fluorescent)
**c** Double amorphous heads

© Springer Nature Switzerland AG 2020
D. Paoli et al., *Atlas of Human Semen Examination*, Trends in Andrology and Sexual Medicine,
https://doi.org/10.1007/978-3-030-39998-6_6

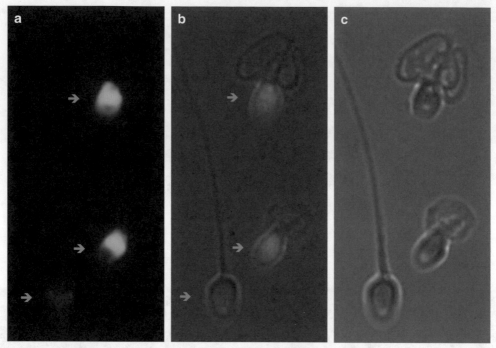

**Fig. 157**  **a, b** ➜ Two spermatozoa with fragmented DNA (fluorescent heads)
➜ Spermatozoon with intact DNA (non-fluorescent head)
**c** Three small heads with small acrosome

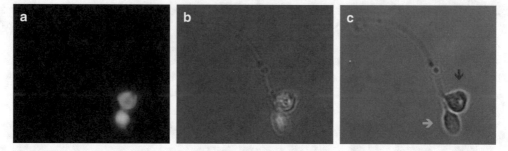

**Fig. 158**  **a** Two heads with fragmented DNA (fluorescent)
**b** Double head (fluorescent)
**c** ➜ Double head with small head, ➜ amorphous head

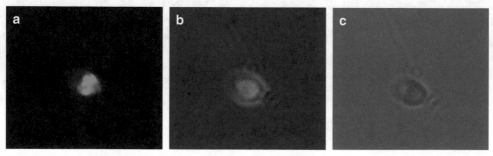

**Fig. 159**  **a, b** Spermatozoon with fragmented DNA (fluorescent head)
**c** Normal head with bent neck

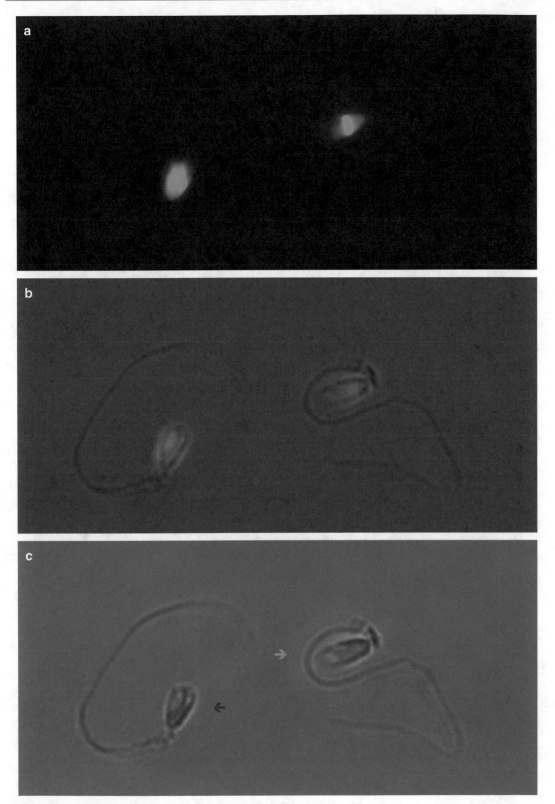

**Fig. 160   a, b** Two spermatozoa with fragmented DNA (fluorescent heads)
**c** ➔ Pyriform head, ➔ Tapered head

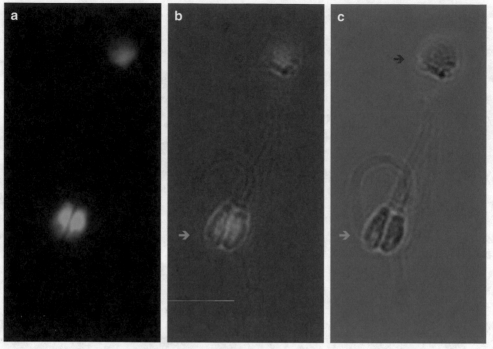

**Fig. 161   a** Three heads with fragmented DNA (fluorescent)
**b** ➔ Double fluorescent head and double tail, ➔ fluorescent head
**c** ➔ Double tapered head and double tail, ➔ amorphous head

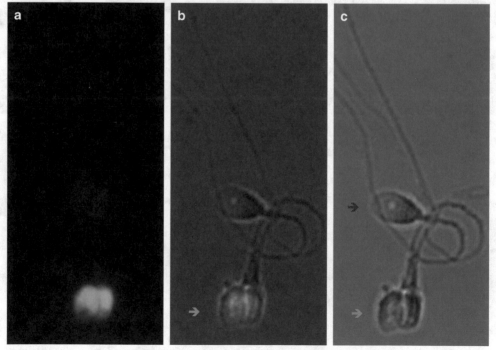

**Fig. 162   a** Two spermatozoa with fragmented DNA (fluorescent heads)
**b, c** ➔ Double head, double tail, ➔ Normal head

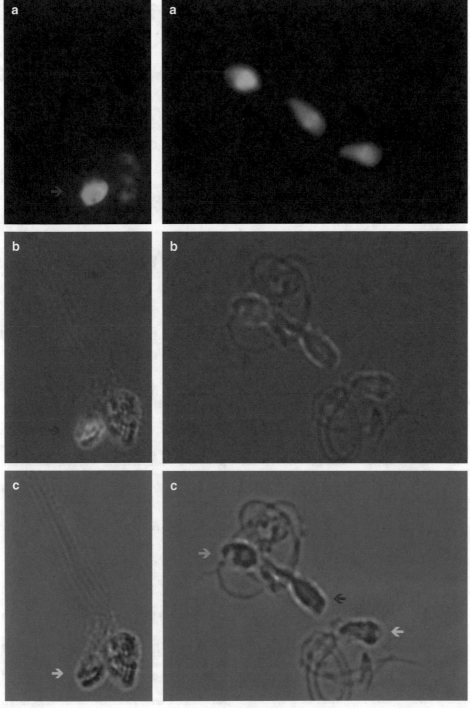

**Fig. 163  a, b →** Spermatozoon with fragmented
DNA (fluorescent
head)
**c →** Amorphous head

**Fig. 164  a, b** Three spermatozoa with
fragmented DNA (fluorescent heads)
**c →** Small head,
**→** Tapered head,
**→** Pyriform head

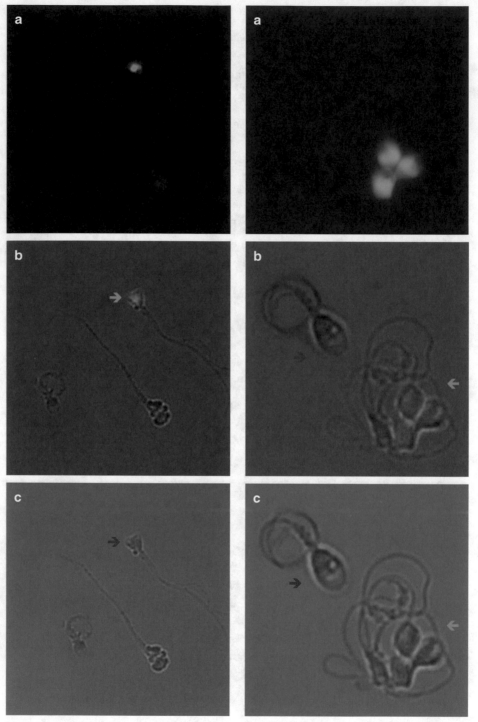

**Fig. 165  a** Head with fragmented DNA
(fluorescent)
**b** ➔ Double head (fluorescent)
**c** ➔ Double small heads and
double tail

**Fig. 166  a** Three heads with fragmented DNA
(fluorescent)
**b, c** ➔ Three fluorescent amorphous
heads,
➔ Non-fluorescent normal head

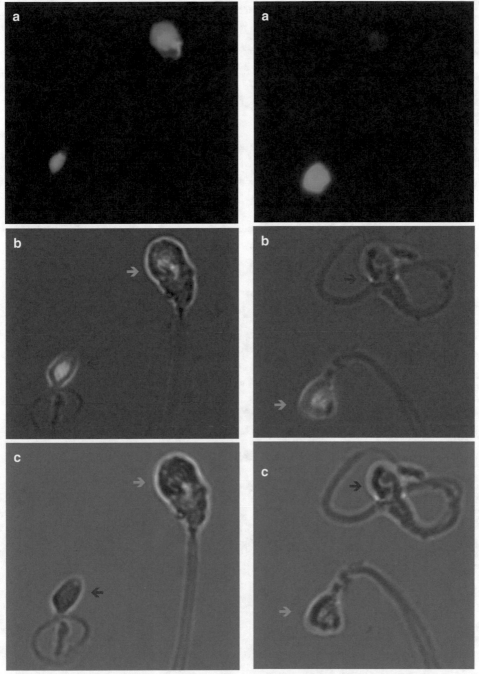

**Fig. 167** **a** Two heads with fragmented DNA
(fluorescent)
**b, c** ➔ Small head and small acrosome,
➔ Double head, double tail

**Fig. 168** **a** Head with fragmented DNA
(fluorescent)
**b** ➔ Double fluorescent head
and double tail,
➔ Non-fluorescent head
**c** ➔ Double amorphous head
and double tail,
➔ Amorphous head

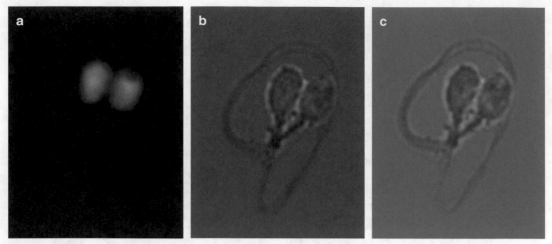

**Fig. 169** **a** Two heads with fragmented DNA (fluorescent)
**b, c** Two amorphous heads

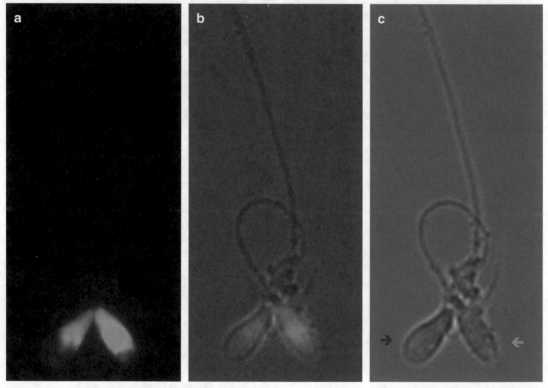

**Fig. 170** **a** Two heads with fragmented DNA (fluorescent)
**b** Double fluorescent head and double tail
**c** Double head, double tail: ➔ Pyriform head, ➔ Tapered head

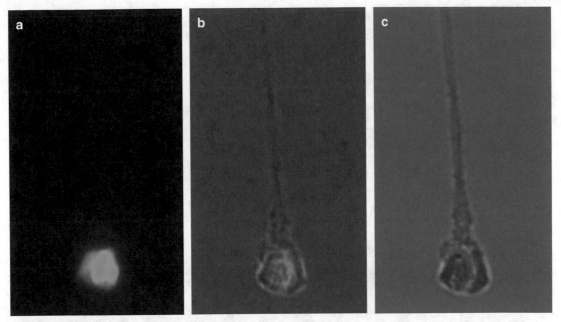

**Fig. 171**   **a** Fluorescent cell
              **b** Double fluorescent head and double tail
              **c** Double amorphous head and double tail

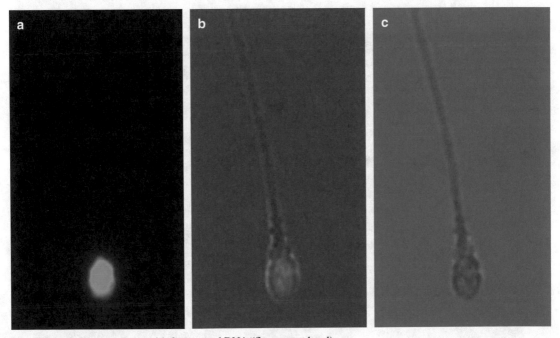

**Fig. 172**   **a, b** Spermatozoon with fragmented DNA (fluorescent head)
              **c** Small head

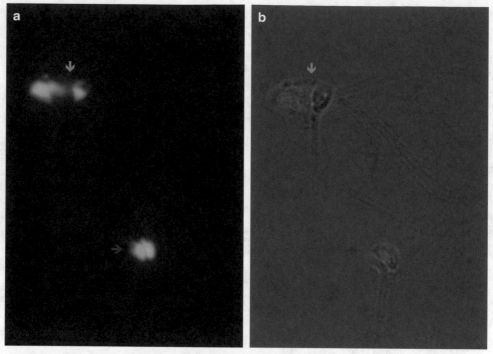

**Fig. 173** a ➜ Three heads with fragmented DNA (fluorescent)
➜ Two heads with fragmented DNA (fluorescent)
b ➜ Three amorphous heads ➜ Double amorphous head and double tail

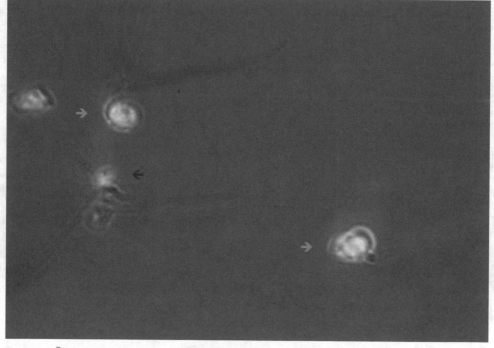

**Fig. 174** ➜ Double heads and double tails with fragmented DNA (fluorescent heads)
➜ Small head with fragmented DNA (fluorescent head)

Printed in the United States
by Baker & Taylor Publisher Services